HOW TO LISTEN SO

MARY HARTLEY is a v
opment coach specializi.
communication. She has considerable experience of
writing on these topics and of presenting work-
shops and courses on aspects of interpersonal
communication and behaviour. As well as contributing to national newspapers and women's and
general-interest magazines, Mary has broadcast on
national and local radio programmes on issues such
as managing anger and coping with stress, and has
acted as consultant for the BBC Learning Zone.
Her books *The Good Stress Guide*, *Managing
Anger at Work*, *Body Language at Work*, *Stress at
Work* and *The Assertiveness Handbook* are all
published by Sheldon Press.

Overcoming Common Problems Series

Selected titles

A full list of titles is available from Sheldon Press,
36 Causton Street, London SW1P 4ST and on our website at
www.sheldonpress.co.uk

Overcoming Common Problems

How to Listen So that People Talk

Mary Hartley

sheldon PRESS

First published in Great Britain in 2006

Sheldon Press
36 Causton Street
London SW1P 4ST

British Library Cataloguing-in-Publication Data
A catalogue record for this book is available from the British Library

ISBN-13: 978–0–85969–969–3
ISBN-10: 0–85969–969–2

1 3 5 7 9 10 8 6 4 2

Typeset by Deltatype Limited, Birkenhead, Merseyside
Printed in Great Britain by
Ashford Colour Press

Contents

1

The importance of listening

The skill of listening

People often assume that listening is easy. After all, they say, it's an activity that we do every day and one that requires no effort. If only that were the case, many problems in communicating with and understanding other people would cease to exist. The truth is that effective listening is a skill that does not come automatically, but it is one that can be learnt and practised.

Listening is the most used and least understood communication skill. In general, we spend 9 per cent of our time writing, 16 per cent reading, 35 per cent talking and 40 per cent listening, yet many of us make little effort to acquire or develop listening skills. We learnt to listen by picking up and imitating the habits of others, who themselves 'picked it up' in a similar way. It is quite likely that many of the listening habits we have picked up are ones that actually block effective communication.

We can all become better listeners. The first step is to recognize that we can learn to listen. We can replace unhelpful habits with practices that encourage understanding and communication.

Why good listening matters

Poor listening is the cause of communication breakdowns in every area of life. Problems need to be understood before they can be solved, instructions need to be taken in before they can be followed, ideas need to be shared and absorbed before they can be evaluated. Ask people what the main causes of difficulties in personal relationships are, and one of the issues that comes up time and time again is lack of listening. Relationships are built, maintained and nurtured by people listening to each other and, conversely, problems develop when we feel that we are not being listened to. When we are not heard, we feel hurt, deflated, let down. Our self-esteem is damaged. If someone does not attend to us and listen to what we are saying, what comes across to us is that we are being discounted, dismissed, rejected. Being listened to fosters our sense of self-worth and lets us know that our thoughts, feelings and ideas are valued. It means that we are taken seriously.

THE IMPORTANCE OF LISTENING

What you will gain from becoming a good listener

If you become a good listener, you will find that your sensitivity to and awareness of other people will increase, leading to improved communication and relationships in all areas of your personal, social and working life. Improved listening will lessen the stress that is caused by frustration and misunderstanding. It will help you to build strong, well-balanced relationships with all the people in your life. It will strengthen your leadership skills and enable you to generate commitment and enthusiasm in others. Best of all, good listening will affirm the value you place on other people and you, in turn, will be recognized and appreciated. As the business guru Tom Peters said, 'Listening is the highest form of courtesy.' When you show interest, understanding and response to someone, you are giving that person a rare and valuable gift.

Exercise: What will you gain?

How will becoming a good listener improve your life? For each of the following suggestions, think of a specific situation in which improved listening skills will make a difference.

I will be able to:	*in this situation:*
communicate more effectively with my partner	_____
communicate more effectively with my children	_____
understand what makes other people tick	_____
be a better friend	_____
be successful at work	_____
understand problems	_____
remember things	_____
take in information more effectively	_____
be a good learner	_____
ask effective and appropriate questions	_____
solve problems	_____
negotiate with others	_____
be a good decision-maker	_____
stay calm in difficult situations	_____
build good relationships	_____
be more confident in social situations	_____

2

handle disagreements	_____
other	_____
other	_____
other	_____

Listening and hearing

Listening is not a natural process, whereas hearing is. If your ears and brain are not damaged, you cannot help but hear sounds of a certain intensity, whether you want to or not. You are not actually listening to the loud music blasting from a passing car, but you cannot help hearing it. Listening, however, is something you choose to do. You can choose to become a good listener and create situations that encourage others to talk openly and confidently, secure in the knowledge that their meaning will be heard and understood. If you choose to listen well, what you engage in is a complicated activity. It involves interpreting and understanding verbal and non-verbal messages, clarifying ambiguous information and encouraging meaningful communication.

Listening is more than a skill – it is an attitude to other people that indicates acceptance and respect. The quality of your listening can either affirm a person's worth and value or undermine it. Take the first step to developing this attribute by acknowledging the import- ance of attentive, effective listening.

Listening and talking

A good listener contributes to the conversation. Effective listening means feeding back to others that their words and message have been understood. It means making responses that promote further communication and understanding. Some of these responses are non- verbal, others are spoken. Listening is not a passive activity – it is, in fact, a two-way process.

> If we were supposed to talk more than we listen,
> we would have two mouths and one ear.
>
> Mark Twain

In other words, we should listen more than we speak, but speaking and responding are important as well.

Exercise: What kind of listener are you?

Think about the kind of listener you are at the moment. Answer the following questions as honestly as you can. If a statement describes your listening attitudes or behaviour on the whole, tick 'Yes', if not, tick 'No'.

		Yes	No
1	I listen without interrupting.	☐	☐
2	I show that I am listening when a speaker is talking.	☐	☐
3	I tend to be easily distracted.	☐	☐
4	I ask questions.	☐	☐
5	I ask a variety of types of questions.	☐	☐
6	I control my mannerisms and body language.	☐	☐
7	When I am having a difficult conversation, I prepare my responses as I am listening.	☐	☐
8	I sometimes finish other people's sentences to show that I understand what they are saying.	☐	☐
9	I check to make sure that I have understood properly.	☐	☐
10	My concentration lapses if the speaker is hard to follow.	☐	☐
11	I don't let my own thoughts interfere with my listening.	☐	☐
12	I think it is up to the speaker to make his or her meaning clear.	☐	☐
13	I find it hard to regulate eye contact with the speaker.	☐	☐
14	I can use a range of responses.	☐	☐
15	I listen for the emotion as well as the words.	☐	☐
16	I often miss the point of what someone is saying.	☐	☐
17	I wait for the speaker to finish before I evaluate what has been said.	☐	☐
18	I reflect back and paraphrase what has been said.	☐	☐
19	I can put aside my own personal needs while I listen.	☐	☐
20	I can't help responding emotionally sometimes.	☐	☐

The answers to this exercise are on page 119.

If you got ten or more right answers, you have a sound basis on which to build your listening skills. Don't worry if you have fewer correct responses – you will be surprised how quickly you can develop good listening habits once you decide to do so.

If you feel that your listening skills are not very good, you are not alone. One study of listening shows that we use only a quarter of our listening potential, only really taking in a quarter of what is said to us. The other three quarters of what we hear is forgotten or misunderstood or not heeded or twisted. Another study of listening effectiveness shows that we tend to forget one third to one half of what we hear within eight hours! Overall, it seems that it is common for us to miss about half of what someone tells us. Many misunderstandings are caused by the fact that, when we speak, we assume that the other person hears what we say when, in fact, it seems that there is very little guarantee that such communication takes place.

Poor listening habits

It is easy to drift into bad listening behaviour without realizing that we are doing so. We get used to interrupting people who say things we disagree with. We find that we switch off when certain people are speaking or jump to conclusions about what someone is going to say. These are habits of listening behaviour. The first step towards replacing poor listening habits with more helpful ones is recognizing the areas in which we could improve.

Exercise: Poor listening habits

1   Use the previous exercise to help you identify any poor listening habits you may have. Tick the appropriate column below to show how often you display this habit. (You might need to ask someone for some feedback to help you answer.)

	Often	Occasionally	Never
Changing the subject inappropriately	☐	☐	☐
Fidgeting	☐	☐	☐
Not offering ideas and opinions	☐	☐	☐
Mentally switching off	☐	☐	☐
Jumping to conclusions	☐	☐	☐
Finishing people's sentences for them	☐	☐	☐

THE IMPORTANCE OF LISTENING

	Often	Occasionally	Never
Listening on the run	☐	☐	☐
Talking too much	☐	☐	☐
Hearing what you want to hear	☐	☐	☐
Selecting what stands out for you	☐	☐	☐
Sneaking a look at the time	☐	☐	☐
Interrupting	☐	☐	☐
Carrying on with other activities	☐	☐	☐
Looking as if there were more important things to do	☐	☐	☐
Moving off before the speaker has finished	☐	☐	☐
Asking a question about something that has just been explained	☐	☐	☐
Changing the topic when the speaker pauses	☐	☐	☐
Looking bored	☐	☐	☐
Thinking about something else	☐	☐	☐
Looking away	☐	☐	☐
Staring into space	☐	☐	☐
Other	☐	☐	☐
Other	☐	☐	☐
Other	☐	☐	☐

2   Now choose the six habits that you would most like to improve.

(a) _____

(b) _____

(c) _____

(d) _____

(e) _____

(f) _____

_____

What makes a good listener?

Good listeners display patience, understanding and empathy. They use a range of interpersonal skills that they deploy with sensitivity and respect. When talking with others, good listeners can establish rapport and get on the same wavelength. They make appropriate eye contact and their body language conveys attention and responsiveness. They listen to the whole person and the whole message, not just to the words that are spoken, and do not allow the message to become distorted by personal bias. They listen actively, making encouraging responses and checking the messages that they receive.

Exercise: Keeping track

As you work on building your listening skills, concentrate on replacing the particular unhelpful habits you have identified with more positive responses. Think of the situations in which you find it hard to listen attentively and set yourself manageable goals for improvement. Keep a record of your progress.

Situation	Unhelpful habit	Goal
e.g. Talking to Jasmine	Not showing interest	Make eye contact

2

Why we don't listen well

Barriers to good listening

Many factors prevent us from listening well. Some of these are external conditions, such as the place in which the conversation happens or our physical state at the time, and some are internal, such as our emotional condition or our feelings about the person with whom we are speaking. Sometimes the difficulty lies with the other person, who intentionally or unintentionally may send unclear or incomplete messages.

The time and the place

Do aspects of this situation sound familiar? It is the end of a long, hard day and you are looking forward to sitting down with a cup of tea or a cold beer and having a relaxing half an hour in front of the television or reading the paper or listening to music or just chilling out. As soon as you sit down, someone bursts in or the phone rings and you hear something like one of the following:

'The washing machine has flooded the kitchen.'
'They're putting the rent up.'
'I want to talk about our relationship.'
'I got suspended from school today.'

When it is the wrong time of day or the wrong moment for you, listening calmly and attentively can be very difficult. Our moods, habits and preferences mean that we are more receptive at some times than at others and, when there is a clash of preferences, then communication suffers. If you like to go to bed early, but your partner likes to chat late at night and brings up significant issues at that time, it is likely that you will find it hard to concentrate on what is said and resent efforts to make you communicate at that time of day. Then your partner will feel frustrated and rejected because you won't talk. Similarly, you might want to hear about your children's day at school as soon as you see them, but they might need to put a little distance between themselves and the day's events before they can talk about it.

Scene: The wrong moment for Jackie
Jackie has brought home a report that she needs to finish by the next morning. She tells the children not to disturb her. She is concentrating on some tricky footnotes when Holly bursts in and says, 'Liam's spoilt my painting on purpose!' Her voice is tearful.
'I'm sure he didn't,' says Jackie distractedly. 'Why don't you do another one?'

Later that week, Jackie wonders why Holly accuses her of not being fair and taking Liam's side in everything.

In the earlier situation, Jackie responded instinctively. She was anxious to get her work finished and so did not pay attention to what Holly was saying. She heard the words, but not the meaning and the emotion behind the words, because in the circumstances she was not able to tune in to Holly's message.

Exercise: The right circumstances

How attentively can you listen and respond in the following circumstances?

	Not very	A little	Hardly at all
While you are driving	☐	☐	☐
While you are reading	☐	☐	☐
While you are writing	☐	☐	☐
When you are tired	☐	☐	☐
On a land line phone	☐	☐	☐
On a mobile phone in public	☐	☐	☐
Travelling on a bus	☐	☐	☐
Travelling on a train	☐	☐	☐
Travelling on a plane	☐	☐	☐
Walking with someone	☐	☐	☐
Watching television	☐	☐	☐
Doing household chores/ maintenance	☐	☐	☐
Late at night	☐	☐	☐
Early in the morning	☐	☐	☐
When you are feeling angry or emotional about something	☐	☐	☐
When you are worried about something	☐	☐	☐
In a noisy bar	☐	☐	☐

9

WHY WE DON'T LISTEN WELL

	Not very	A little	Hardly at all
In a noisy restaurant	☐	☐	☐
In a noisy office	☐	☐	☐
When you are in a hurry	☐	☐	☐
When the phone keeps ringing	☐	☐	☐
While you are cooking	☐	☐	☐
Playing a computer game	☐	☐	☐
When you need to concentrate on something	☐	☐	☐
When music is playing	☐	☐	☐
When something is on your mind	☐	☐	☐
Other	☐	☐	☐
Other	☐	☐	☐
Other	☐	☐	☐

Being prepared

You have identified some of your own preferences, but of course not everyone will share them. You might find it helpful to identify how other people communicate in different circumstances. This will make you aware of the situations in which the people you interact with are likely to become communicative. With some people in your life, you can base your observations on your personal experience of communicating with them. For example, you will know the individuals in your private and professional life who are happy to receive phone calls at home or late in the evening and you will know those who like to be called only at work or only before a certain time of night. You know the friends who like chatting at home and those who don't open up a lot when they are at home, but will bring up important matters when they are out for a meal or a drink. You may have to experiment a little with people you don't know well, but, once you are alert to this aspect of communication, you will soon notice others' personal preferences.

However, preferences are not hard and fast guidelines. We are all subject to changing moods and feelings. Sometimes a certain time and place works, at other times they don't. Sometimes significant conversations can take place in the most unexpected circumstances, while situations that you think will be conducive to positive communication do not produce the expected results. For example, you might have arranged a get-together over a drink or dinner, hoping to discuss a particular issue, but somehow it doesn't get

10

going and one or the other of you feels frustrated, but when you are just driving to the shops with no intention of having a significant conversation, you find that you talk easily and really listen to what the other says. As a good listener, you will be prepared to give the appropriate level of attention to the other person whatever the circumstances.

Exercise: The right time and place

Choose six people with whom you would like to communicate more effectively. Identify the kinds of circumstances in which they are most responsive.

	Person	Place	Time
1			
2			
3			
4			
5			
6			

When it's the wrong time

Sometimes you know that you are not going to be able to listen attentively because the time and place are wrong for you. In these circumstances, it is best to say so and postpone the conversation. It is impossible to be focused and empathetic if you are just not feeling up to it. This applies to both personal conversations and communication at work. When you are unable to pay full attention, for whatever reason, you could find yourself giving responses that you later regret.

Scene: Vikram goes for the right moment

Vikram is looking forward to meeting a friend at lunchtime. Just before lunch, his line manager starts to discuss Vikram's role in the forthcoming reorganization of the department. Vikram hears what his manager is saying and, wanting to show his cooperation, nods at one or two points, then realizes that he is not listening as closely as he wants to.

'I really want to discuss this with you,' Vikram says, 'but I've got a lunchtime appointment that is on my mind at the moment. When would be a good time?'

Of course, there is an element of risk in telling someone you don't want to talk or cutting across a conversation someone has begun, but acknowledging that you are not able to concentrate on it properly at that moment is actually the respectful and responsible thing to do. It indicates that you take the matter seriously and wish to give the subject and person the full attention they deserve. Also, this behaviour sends a message to the other person that when someone is about to start a significant conversation, it is helpful to all concerned to ask if it is a good time to do so.

Physical barriers

Comfort matters

Communication is affected by the physical conditions in which it takes place. You may find it difficult to listen to someone speaking if the room is too cold or too hot or if there is a lot of background noise. Seating or standing arrangements may present a barrier if, for example, you have to strain to hear someone who is placed at an uncomfortable distance from you.

Your own physical state can interfere with your conversation. You might be in the middle of a conversation and realize that you are getting very hungry or your headache is getting worse.

If you find that physical conditions make it hard for you to stay focused on what someone is saying, do what you can to make the situation better. If the arrangement of a room makes it difficult for you to listen, make appropriate changes. Move your chair closer to the other person or choose a chair that is at the same height. If there is a desk between you, try moving so that you are both on the same side of it. Move away from noisy equipment or machinery. Turn lights up or down as appropriate. If you are hungry or have a headache, do whatever is usually helpful for you – have a drink of water, take a tablet or do a tension-relieving exercise. If you don't do something about the distraction, you are likely to end up focusing on that rather than on the other person. Removing physical barriers and distractions will encourage more effective listening and better communication.

If you are stuck in difficult circumstances you cannot change, try to tune out the distraction. Channel your concentration and energy towards the other person and focus on listening.

Information overload

We can only take in so much information at a time. When someone talks for too long or gives us too much information, we tune out and reject what we cannot deal with. We tend to listen most attentively at the beginning and end of a lengthy message, which is why we remember the introduction and conclusion of a long talk and probably just the first and last few directions of an instruction that consists of ten steps.

Gender issues

Recent research has come up with a reason for men sometimes switching off when they are listening to women. It is to do with the different qualities of male and female voices and the effort it takes to listen to each. Female voices are more complicated than men's, with a larger range of soundwaves. They have a singsong musical quality that makes the natural melody of speech more pronounced. This means that female voices are harder to listen to than male voices, requiring more concentration.

Psychological barriers

Your personal filters and worldview

We all view the world we inhabit through our own filters. We perceive and interpret everything we experience via our individual consciousness, and our view is shaped by our whole background: our past experiences, education, personality, needs and motives. When your worldview, beliefs and values are different from someone else's, you may find that this forms a barrier to communication. It can be hard to understand and empathize with someone whose approach to life is very different from our own and whose views and attitudes we don't share.

In these circumstances, we need to make a conscious effort to listen with empathy and objectivity. This does not mean that we have to agree with what is being said, but, for the time that we are listening, we have to suspend our own attitudes and pay attention to the other person.

Listening to someone whose whole belief and value system is at odds with your own is very different from tuning in to someone who is expressing a point of view with which you disagree, but whose fundamental attitudes you share.

Scene: Different values
Marsha is telling Jane about a stressful shopping trip she had with her daughter.

'She insisted on this particular pair of jeans,' says Marsha, 'and she just wouldn't consider any of the cheaper options! So I had no choice but to fork out for them, and that's completely maxed out my credit card. I'm worried about how I'm going to get through the month. I wake up early trying to do sums in my head. It's really getting to me.'

Jane cannot understand the way that Marsha handles money. Marsha spends a lot and lives on credit, which is not Jane's way at all, and seems to encourage her children to have the same attitude. As a friend in whom Marsha is confiding, Jane has to make the effort to suppress her instinctive disapproval and concentrate on listening to how Marsha is feeling. Of course she will be able to give her point of view and move into a discussion of the situation, if she wishes, but a good listener makes the effort to understand the person speaking before evaluating or judging what is said.

Exercise: Be aware of your own beliefs and attitudes

Draw a circle around any of the following subjects about which you have strongly held beliefs or opinions.

money	religion	sexual behaviour	bringing up children
politics	family	sport	entertainment

Other

Other

Other

Being aware of your own beliefs and values will help you to listen objectively. You can tell yourself, 'OK, what is being said doesn't reflect my own view, but I can put my attitude aside for the moment and concentrate on seeing things from the other person's view.'

Making assumptions

No matter how unbiased we think we are, bias and assumptions are built into the way that we perceive the world. We have to be like this if we are to make any sense of what we see and hear. Communication is eased by our ability to decipher the variety and number of signals that we receive. We make instant judgements about people based on their appearance and behaviour and instant assessments of situations based on our experience and knowledge of the world. If you enter a building marked 'Convent' and see a group of women wearing nuns' habits, you will probably make the reasonable assumption that the women are nuns. If you are in a bar in the evening and see a group of women wearing nuns' habits, you will probably not jump to the same conclusion, but think that they are more likely to be with a fancy dress or hen party.

What you need to check is that your assumptions are not based solely on your own subjective opinions. If you make assumptions about a person, you have already decided what that person will say, so, instead of listening attentively, you automatically dismiss what is said or select aspects of the conversation that fit your preconceived ideas. You look for evidence to support your ideas and don't hear anything the person says that contradicts them.

Scene: Faith jumps to conclusions

Faith is listening to her friend's plans for taking a year out of work.

'I'd like to go and work for an aid agency,' Tara says, 'maybe in Africa, but Kerry's idea is that we do bar work here to get some money and then do a round-the-world trip.'

'That's settled then,' says Faith. 'You'll do what Kerry says, as usual.'

Faith has assumed that Tara will fall in with Kerry's plans. She does not focus on what Tara has revealed about her own preference, nor pick up on the opportunity and implied invitation to discuss the matter.

Hearing what we expect to hear

There will be some people you don't listen to because you already know what they are going to say. You are so familiar with their thoughts, attitudes and preoccupations that, when they open their mouths to speak, you hardly bother to tune in.

15

Scene: Knowing what someone will say
Callum says to his father, 'I was called in to the Head of Year's office today and . . .'
Terry explodes: 'I'm sick and tired of you getting into trouble! What was it this time?'
'I wasn't in trouble. She wanted to ask me to go in for a competition, that's all. I thought you'd be pleased. I should have known!' He storms out and slams the door.

As Callum has been in a lot of trouble at school recently, Terry has become programmed to anticipate bad news. If he had paid more attention to the way that Callum was speaking, he would have realized that Callum's tone of voice and facial expression indicated that something good had happened.

Hearing what we want to hear and not hearing what we don't want to hear

Sometimes we hear not what the person actually says, but what we want him or her to have said. One way in which we do this is by picking up on little words, phrases, facial expressions and gestures and removing them from the context of the whole conversation so that the speaker's intention is twisted and distorted to suit our needs. When we don't like what we are hearing, we can put up a kind of road block to stop the actual message from getting through.

Scene: Leaving the nest
All Maggie's children have left home except her son James. Maggie likes having James around – he is good fun, easy to live with and she enjoys his company.
On his way out one evening, James says, 'Oh, by the way, I looked at a flat today.'
Maggie's stomach gives a little lurch. 'Oh yes?' she says guardedly.
'One of those in the new development,' James goes on. 'It's ridiculously expensive, of course, and the parking's not ideal, but I really liked it. Dan's coming to have a look at it tonight. If he feels the same as I do, we'll go ahead. You'll love it – state-of-the-art kitchen and a great bathroom!'
Later that evening, Maggie says to her husband, 'James said something about one of those new flats, but they're really expensive and he wouldn't be able to park, so I think we'll be stuck with him for a bit longer!'
Maggie didn't hear what James was saying. The whole

message conveys that he and Dan will probably move into the flat in spite of the drawbacks, that it is expensive and the parking is not good, but Maggie does not want to acknowledge this. She does not draw from James' words the fact that he is ready to leave home and if he doesn't go ahead with this flat, it is likely that he will look for another one. She does not hear the way that he lets her know that he is not excluding her from his life either – Maggie's emotional needs act as a barrier to her listening.

Being prejudiced towards someone

Being prejudiced in someone's favour can also prevent attentive listening. When we like or admire people, it is possible for us to be ready to respond positively to whatever they say. It may not even be actual liking that influences us – we can be biased in someone's favour by such factors as coming from the same town, having gone to the same school or supporting the same football team. Sometimes just one or two qualities that we like in someone have the knock-on effect of causing us to judge the whole person in a favourable way – a reaction that is called 'the halo effect'.

Scene: Damian and the halo effect

Damian is looking for someone to act as temporary team leader in his department, with the possibility of this becoming permanent. He has observed Sally working and likes the way that she deals with customers. She is popular with her colleagues and is good at diffusing conflict.

At the interview, Damian asks Sally to describe how she would handle a member of staff who will not keep to deadlines. She says, 'I would understand the problem, because I'm not great at time management myself, so what I would do is ...' Damian nods approvingly as Sally talks about the importance of communication and how she would first find out why the person had such a difficulty.

Damian's admiration of Sally's interpersonal skills means that he is already inclined to favour her and so he does not pick up any negative points in Sally's application, such as her statement that she is not a good time manager.

Being prejudiced against someone

It can be difficult to listen properly when we are prejudiced against someone. Sometimes we are hardly aware that we are prejudiced, but it is often the case that we are distracted and misled by aspects of people's appearance, personality or background that incline us to regard them unfavourably before we listen to what they have to say.

Scene: The trouble with the younger generation
Barry looks at the clock as Scott comes through the door and suppresses a sigh of irritation. No doubt about it, the younger generation is not half as meticulous about timekeeping as his has always been. They have different standards of dress, too. Barry unconsciously straightens his tie as he regards Scott's baggy jeans and earrings.

'If it's not rushing you too much,' he says in a heavy attempt at jocularity, 'we could have a word about the Wilson order.'

'Sure.' Scott saunters over and pulls up a chair.

Barry moves behind his desk and keeps his back straight. He has no time for the lounging attitude people like Scott seem to find appropriate.

Exercise: Prejudice and listening

I find it easy to pay unbiased attention to someone:

	Always	Sometimes	Never
much younger than me	☐	☐	☐
much older than me	☐	☐	☐
of a different culture	☐	☐	☐
of a different race	☐	☐	☐
of a different sexual orientation	☐	☐	☐
of a lower level of education	☐	☐	☐
of different professional standing	☐	☐	☐
whose voice I dislike	☐	☐	☐
from a different social background	☐	☐	☐
with strong religious beliefs	☐	☐	☐
with religious beliefs different from mine	☐	☐	☐
who swears	☐	☐	☐
who uses racist terminology	☐	☐	☐
who uses sexist terminology	☐	☐	☐
with different political views	☐	☐	☐
other	☐	☐	☐
other	☐	☐	☐

'We're losing money over this order,' he says. 'It's just not happening quickly enough. There's a bottleneck somewhere and we have to track it down.'

'Yeah, right,' says Scott.

Barry tries not to wince too visibly.

'I have been thinking about this,' says Scott. He rocks back on his chair and picks at his fingernails. 'It could be in despatch.'

Barry frowns. 'Sounds very unlikely to me. In my experience, that's always been the most efficient department.'

Scott shrugs and goes back to his desk. He has checked his facts and he knows that he is right, but he also knows that whatever he says, Barry won't hear.

Barry does not like the appearance and behaviour of Scott's generation and this colours the way in which he communicates with Scott. He is not able to listen attentively to him and immediately discounts what he says.

Knowing and acknowledging your own areas of prejudice will alert you to the importance of setting aside your preconceptions and paying close attention.

Emotional triggers

Our emotional reactions can create a barrier and prevent us from listening. Being in the grip of strong feelings is overwhelming and makes us unable to think and react in a rational way. When something is said that triggers feelings of anger or hurt or fear, we may flare up and hit back. Our automatic defensiveness prevents us from taking in the whole message and, instead of listening calmly, we retaliate and attack the other person or instinctively defend or excuse ourselves. This is a common reaction in situations where we are being criticized or think that we are. However, we need to manage and control such a response to prevent a barrier being formed.

Many of us find that we have emotional responses to certain words or phrases. These expressions trigger a reaction that can be so strong as to make us unable to hear what is actually being said. The emotion triggered could be support, anger, envy, suspicion, disapproval, warmth, fear, guilt or whatever feeling it is that is closely linked with that word in your mind.

Value-laden words

The words that act as triggers may be ones associated with our values and beliefs and refer to matters about which we have strong, ingrained feelings.

Scene: The stay-at-home mother

Lisa does not do paid work outside the home. She chooses to devote her time to caring for her small children and running a comfortable home. For Lisa, this is a way of life that reflects her values.

Lisa meets Jenny at a friend's house and finds her to be enjoyable and interesting company. Jenny is encouraging Lisa to join the local theatre group.

Jenny says, 'They're a great bunch of people, all ages and types, some stay-at-home mums like you . . .'

Lisa feels that this phrase demeans her chosen role in life. Lisa resents what she sees as the implication that she leads a passive life and feels angry and uncomfortable. From this moment on, she tunes Jenny out and does not really listen to what she is saying.

Exercise: Your emotional triggers

Do you have a distinct emotional reaction – positive or negative – to any of the following phrases?

justice	immigrant	stay-at-home mum	family values	modern art
entrepreneur		political correctness		fee-paying schools
National Health Service		single mum		taking drugs
equal opportunities		positive discrimination		thirty-somethings
homeless people	gap-year students		binge drinkers	

other

other

other

Words that reflect your present priorities

We are all alert to words and phrases that refer to our current preoccupations. If you are pregnant, your ears will pick up references to pregnancy that you may well not have noticed otherwise; if you are planning a holiday in a certain country, you will hear references to that country; if you are thinking of buying a new car, it may well seem that everyone is suddenly talking about and driving the particular model you are keen on. This is because your mind informs your brain to notice references to what interests it and filter out redundant information. This is all part of the way in which we select information.

Unfortunately, this selection process can get in the way of accurate listening, causing you to be so focused on the part of what is being said that interests you at the moment that you do not pay full attention to the whole of the message. Of course, unlike your response to value-laden words, when your interest in the particular subject has passed, the words will not arouse the same response.

Scene: The hooded top
The school at which Brett teaches is on a drive to enforce wearing of the correct school uniform. Brett takes this very seriously and is pleased with the success of the campaign. This morning, a junior teacher says to him, 'I might be worrying about nothing, but one of the Year 9 girls whose name I don't know, she's got short red hair and is wearing a hooded top, well, she . . .'

Brett explodes, 'They all know they're not allowed to wear those tops! I'll send a message that she has to report for detention!' He strides off.

Brett's preoccupation with the uniform rule has led to him not listening to what his colleague has to say. His lack of attention means that his colleague feels snubbed and frustrated because she has not been able to draw to Brett's attention what might be an important matter.

Exercise: My triggers

Which people and situations cause you to respond angrily and defensively, so that you do not really listen to what they say?

Person to whom I react emotionally or overreact   *Issue*
e.g. My partner   Comments about
                                                     my weight

1 _____

2 _____

3 _____

4 _____

5 _____

6 _____

The desire to protect

The desire to protect yourself might lead to you not hearing anything that might threaten your sense of security and well-being. Equally, the desire to protect someone else might cause you to be unable to acknowledge the person's feelings of, say, anxiety or unhappiness.

> *Scene: Mel wants it to be all right*
> Lorraine is going on a trekking holiday – something she has always wanted to do. She won't know anyone else in the party. Just before the departure date, she says to her older sister, 'I suppose it's too late for me to drop out?'
> Mel says, 'Why would you want to do that? You've been looking forward to it!'
> Lorraine says, 'I suppose so. It's just that I will be going by myself.'
> 'It'll be fine!' says Mel heartily. 'You'll have a great time!'
> Mel's desire to make everything all right for her sister means that she doesn't want to hear any expressions of doubt or apprehension. Her response does not encourage Lorraine to communicate how she is feeling.

Exercise: Emotional responses

What is your instinctive, emotional response to each of the following statements?

'They are being horrible to me at school. No one will let me play with them.'
'We're so proud of Annie! All top grades in her exams!'
'I'm feeling really low and depressed.'
'I think we should have separate holidays this year.'
'I have to tell you – I'm leaving Tom. The children are going to stay with him.'
'I've had a substantial lottery win!'
'I've been promoted. More money, bigger car, the lot.'

Some of the emotions you experience might be:

pleasure	anger	protectiveness	fear	resentment
envy	sympathy	disapproval	impatience	delight
support	anxiety	interest	relief	impatience

Words/use of language

Language is a means of communication, but it can create a barrier. If someone uses words or phrases that are unfamiliar to you or you do not understand, the process of listening becomes more complicated. Not only do you need to ask for clarification, but there are also issues concerning the nature and intention of this particular use of language. The assumption that the listener is familiar with the terms being used may be justified or unjustified.

Language can be used deliberately to exclude the person listening. Certain types of slang or jargon have this function, creating a sense that the individuals who understand and use it belong to a certain group and those to whom it is unfamiliar are not part of this group and are not in the know.

Distorted thinking

Some kinds of distorted thinking can affect the way that we listen to each other. You may have particular patterns of thoughts and reactions that cause you to misinterpret what people say because you have become programmed to respond in a certain way. For example, it could be that you have a tendency to see only the negative aspect of situations or you tend to think that you are being criticized. Often the reason for skewed reactions such as these is low self-esteem. Sometimes our self-image and feelings about ourselves lead us to hear messages in a distorted way

> *Scene: Debbie hears implied criticism*
> Debbie and Rob are discussing the party that they are arranging for her parents' golden wedding anniversary.
> 'I'm thinking we should get a catering company to do the food,' says Rob. 'It would be far less hassle for you and you'd have more time to relax and socialize.'
> 'Don't you think I'm capable of doing the food?' says Debbie.
> Debbie's low self-esteem makes her hear only the first part of what Rob says and she chooses to hear it as criticism. She takes Rob's suggestion as a slur on her cooking abilities, which is not at all what Rob intended.

Another way of responding that shuts off communication is retreating and clamming up. When we hear something that flicks on the raw, we sometimes refuse to listen or enter into a dialogue. We do the equivalent of what children do when they put their hands over their ears.

Scene: Maeve switches off
Maeve is very weight-conscious. She thinks that she is too heavy and she is sensitive to references about body shape or size.

Maeve and a few friends are slumped in front of the television watching a film award ceremony. They comment on the celebrities' outfits and play a game of giving each one a mark out of ten. One of her friends says of a certain movie star, 'Oh, that dress is totally wrong for her. It makes her look really fat.'

Those words ring in Maeve's head, although the comment was not in the least directed at her. She does not hear or attend to the rest of the conversation.

Being negative

A negative approach to life can prevent us from listening carefully. Instead of hearing the whole message, we focus on one aspect of it and twist what is said to fit our pessimistic attitude.

Scene: Maya makes it negative
Maya's tutor says to her, 'This is a good essay. What you need to do to get a higher mark is to include more references and examples.'

Maya tells her friend, 'She said my essay was hopeless because there weren't enough examples.'

Maya is so ready to tune into negative comments that she does not hear the message being conveyed here. Look at the way she discounts the word 'good' and replaces it with 'hopeless' and does not take in the advice about how to get a higher mark, seeing it instead as a criticism.

Early experiences and messages about listening

When you were growing up, were you aware of people listening to each other? Did people listen to you? Traditional ideas about children being seen and not heard still flourish in different guises. In conversations between adults and children, it can happen that the adults do most of the talking and pay only lip-service to the notion of listening to children. If you were not listened to, appreciated and acknowledged, you may not have developed the habit of communicating and engaging with people.

Some aspects of our upbringing and education do not foster good listening. As pupils and students, we are often required to listen for longer periods of time than we can manage, the result being that we get into the habit of switching off. Another way we cope is by developing the techniques of being able, when challenged, to repeat word for word what has just been said without any idea of its real meaning.

Some unhelpful messages about listening

'It's rude to ask questions.'
'Don't listen to him.'
'Don't pay any attention to that.'
'Pretend you haven't heard.'
'I'll just ignore that.'
'If you ask, you don't get.'
'Don't talk back.'
'Ignorance is bliss.'

Exercise: Barriers you have experienced

Can you identify occasions on which you have experienced barriers to your ability to listen?

Cause of interference	*Occasion*
Physical conditions	_____
Subject matter of conversation	_____
Category of person	_____
Being biased or prejudiced	_____
Values and biases	_____
Making assumptions	_____
Words or phrases	_____
Distorted thinking	_____
Responding emotionally	_____
Past experience	_____

Overcoming barriers to good listening

All the obstacles to attentive listening that we have discussed can be overcome. Once you have identified potential barriers, you can minimize their effect. You can deal with physical barriers by removing them or lessening their impact and you can deal with emotional and psychological ones by mentally distancing yourself from them. You can learn skills, such as reflecting and responding, that help you to listen with an open mind and learn to manage your emotional state so that you are receptive to the speaker. You can find out how to encourage people to respond and develop what they are saying.

Developing listening skills will help you to:

- hear the whole of what someone says;
- check that you have heard and understood;
- keep an open mind;
- overcome bias;
- avoid jumping to conclusions;
- not presume that you know what someone is thinking or feeling;
- evaluate what you hear;
- encourage the person to continue.

3

Tuning in to the other person

Active listening

Active listening is a phrase used to describe a cluster of skills that focus on the circular process of understanding and interpreting what someone is saying, feeding back your perceptions, asking questions and encouraging the development of the conversation. Listening actively means not just attending to what is being said but also making the right choices about how to respond. You will find that when you make conscious decisions about how to listen, the quality of your communication improves dramatically as people are encouraged to talk more purposefully and openly. As we have seen, the skills of attending, understanding and reflecting do not always come naturally, but they can be learnt. Listening is a complicated process and to do it effectively demands discipline and concentration, but remember, the rewards are great, for everyone concerned.

Create the right climate

The right listening climate is not necessarily one that is planned. Given the right circumstances of place and time and readiness on both sides to talk and listen, valuable communication can just happen. Often, though, it needs bit of help.

Understanding the purpose

There is a reason behind every conversation we have. We want to give or receive information or ask for help or advice or entertain or be entertained or express our feelings about something. Breakdowns in communication can occur when the point of the conversation is not acknowledged by the participants. If one or more gets it wrong, you may find that you are speaking at cross-purposes, to the frustration of all concerned.

What people may want from a conversation

For example, they may want to:

- receive or give information;
- unload feelings;

- entertain or be entertained;
- affirm a relationship;
- deepen a relationship;
- understand the other person better;
- exchange confidences;
- reach an agreement;
- clear the air;
- make one's point of view clear.

Scene: Guy doesn't get the point
Ashley has had a bad day at work. Over a drink, he tells Guy about how difficult this particular client has been and how he just about managed to sort it out and then his manager got on his case about that incident the other day, asking why he hadn't had the report yet, although he ought to know that Ashley has been doing two people's jobs . . .

Ashley pauses for breath and Guy says, 'You know, mate, you're wasted in that place. Why don't you sort out your CV and get in touch with a recruitment agency?'

'Whatever,' says Ashley. He feels deflated and thinks that Guy isn't on his wavelength.

Guy has not recognized the purpose of this conversation. Ashley needs to let off steam and unload his frustration and for Guy to listen sympathetically and understand his feelings. If Guy understood what kind of conversation Ashley wanted, he could have chosen a different way of responding.

Make the contract

Setting boundaries

To listen attentively, you have to be comfortable with the time and the place. You may not like communicating on a personal level at work or in public or in the presence of people you don't know well. You may find it hard to pay attention if you are sitting too close to or too far away from the other person or in any of the circumstances we discussed earlier. Just remember to set the contract at the beginning of the conversation and make adjustments if the physical conditions change.

Scene: Stating a boundary
Susie and Liz are having a cappuccino together and discussing

Susie's difficult relationship with her in-laws. Liz is listening attentively and is totally focused on what Susie is saying.

A friend comes over to join them. Susie doesn't mind continuing what she was saying, but Liz feels uncomfortable. She finds the presence of a third person distracting and, in these circumstances, feels inhibited from contributing her own personal responses to the discussion.

As Susie pauses, Liz says, 'I feel that we still have loads to say on this subject. Let's carry on with it when I've had time to digest everything you've said.'

You need to be comfortable with the subject matter as well as the circumstances. Sometimes the precise nature of a conversation is flagged up at the beginning, when someone says, for example, 'Wait till I tell you about what Jay did yesterday!' or 'There's something on my mind. I think Toby is having an affair'. In these circumstances, you can decide if you want to hear what will be said. If you do not feel comfortable with the subject under discussion, it is best to say so. You could say something like, 'You know, I'm not happy talking about Jay/Toby' or 'I don't think I'm the right person to listen to this'. It is better to be open at the beginning than continue with the conversation as, if you allow it to take its course, your discomfort will soon become apparent.

If in the course of a conversation the talk switches to an area you don't want to visit, you have some options. Depending on the circumstances, you could:

- finish the conversation;
- at a suitable point, change the subject;
- disclose your discomfort with the topic.

Getting it going

You may have had the experience of wanting to talk about something, but the right moment for raising it just not materializing. You end up feeling frustrated and dissatisfied.

When you are tuned in to someone's way of behaving and communicating, you pick up the verbal and non-verbal signs that indicate there is something on that person's mind. In these circumstances, a good listener will give the person an opportunity to speak about whatever it is. Often all it takes is for you, the listener, to nudge the conversational door open just a little, giving the speaker a choice as to whether or not to continue.

Opening the door

There are some short phrases that can be used to offer the person a chance to talk. 'Is there something on your mind?' or 'There seems to be something on your mind' are an indication of your sense that there is something that the person would like to say and you are ready to listen. You might just get a shrug and a dismissive reply. If you want to continue to encourage, though, it is a good idea to briefly describe what makes you think that there is something the person might want to share. A description of the person's behaviour or body language works here, but make sure that your tone of voice is quite neutral. You are describing, not challenging or accusing. Something like, 'Well, OK, but you came in frowning and went straight to your room, which you don't normally do', followed by 'Care to talk about it?' is likely to have an encouraging effect.

Scene: Sue invites Josie to talk

Sue's daughter has spent the afternoon at her friend's house.
  'Did you have a good time?' asks Sue.
  Josie shrugs and says, 'It was all right.'
Sue hears that Josie's voice is subdued and sees that her facial expression is tense. She would like Josie to talk to her about it. Sue doesn't pursue the subject right away, having learnt from experience that Josie just clams up if she feels that she is being questioned. Josie is quiet for the rest of the evening. Sue makes her a mug of hot chocolate, her favourite, and says casually, 'You're not as chatty as usual. Anything you can tell me about this afternoon?'
  Josie starts to talk about the quarrel she had with her friend. Sue's phrase gives Josie a bit of encouragement to speak without making her feel under pressure. Sue uses a broad expression that is quite neutral and does not impose Sue's own ideas as to what might have happened on the conversation.

Some phrases to open the door

You could try the following:

  'Something on your mind?'
  'You're looking pleased! Anything to tell me?'
  'I've got time, if you feel like talking.'
  'Would you like to talk about it?'
  'Something's wrong – come on.'

Being present

Another way of opening a door is just by paying attention to someone. Being available in circumstances that will encourage someone to talk can lead to positive communication. This may mean that you make changes to your routine or engineer events so that you synchronize the availability and desire of you both to talk and listen. Tune in to a person's preferences for time and place, as we discussed earlier. If you are present and paying attention in these circumstances, you can use one of the door-openers listed above or just be silent and leave it up to the other to respond to your receptive mode. If you are never or rarely there when people are in the mood to talk, you will never hear what they have to say. So, for example, if someone at home likes to talk about the day or what has been going on as soon as he or she is through the door, you could adapt your pattern of behaviour to be ready to listen to them then. So, instead of being in the middle of household or personal activities or watching television or playing a computer game or catching up on e-mails, you could decide just to be available for the person. It need not be for a long period of time – ten minutes may be enough. It doesn't matter if the person does not always want to talk or is sometimes quiet or abrupt. The likelihood is that your attending presence will promote communication and you may find you establish a routine that makes it easy for conversation to develop.

Closing the door

Some expressions successfully shut down any chance of meaningful communication. Even though they may be well-meaning, they cut across the speaker's needs and feelings and discourage further discussion.

Some phrases that close the door

These include:

> 'Cheer up, it may never happen.'
> 'Oh well, never mind.'
> 'There's no point in talking about it.'
> 'That's all there is to be said on the matter.'
> 'Don't feel so sorry for yourself.'
> 'It will seem better in the morning.'

Old sayings such as 'Worse things happen at sea' and 'It will all come out in the wash' are intended to be comforting, but sound as if you are dismissing the person's feelings.

Tune in to the other person

The next step to becoming a good listener is to focus on the other person. Listening is not about you, it is about someone else. This means giving your physical and mental attention to the speaker and giving the other person physical and psychological space to communicate his or her own story and feelings. It means giving and receiving information ('information' covers the whole range of communication – thoughts, feelings, ideas, jokes, observations, anecdotes and so on) and letting the other person or people know that you are actively listening and participating and tuned in to their presence and words.

Putting aside your own needs

This is a crucial aspect of good listening. For the time being, you have to suspend your own thoughts, needs, impulses. This means that you have to forget all the things that are on your mind and, for as long as you are listening, suppress your own need to be heard. You have to check your instinctive responses and judgements and not allow them to prevent you from giving full attention to the speaker.

Scene: Gill doesn't tune in
Julie sits at the kitchen table, cradling the coffee mug in her hands. Its warmth is comforting and she feels herself calm down a little. She fights the urge to have a cigarette.

Gill pushes across the biscuit tin. 'Go on, have one.'

'I couldn't. I'm too upset to eat anything. We've just had a huge row.'

Gill's eyes widen in sympathy. 'What happened?'

Julie takes a deep breath. She'd come straight round to Gill's as soon as Josh had stormed out.

'Well,' she begins, 'it all started because I said I wouldn't go to the firm's annual dinner.'

'Where are they having it?' asks Gill. 'I've been landed with finding a place for ours.'

Julie feels that the flow of her story has been a little interrupted, but says, 'At the Foxenden Hotel. Anyway, I said it had been so difficult for me last year, not knowing anyone.'

'It's awful when that happens, isn't it,' said Gill. 'I hate it when they all make jokes about work and you don't understand them. That's what happens whenever I meet Ray in that wine bar near his office. Especially that bloke from accounts – you know, the one he had the row with that time.'

'The thing is,' Julie goes on, 'he really took it personally, and he said that I'm not supporting him in his career.'

Gill has left the table and is unloading the dishwasher. Julie carries on speaking to her back.

'That really got me, because it's so unfair and when I told him how I felt he said . . .'

'Damn! This plate's cracked. One of the good ones, too. Sorry – go on. Where were you?'

'Oh, it doesn't matter. I'll tell you some other time.'

Gill is unable to forget her own concerns and preoccupations. All her responses twist the conversation round to herself and what is going on in her life. She hears the words that Julie speaks, but, because she cannot set aside her own self, her responses show that she is not tuned in to Julie's needs and feelings.

Being emotionally ready

Sometimes your state of mind and immediate situation can have a negative effect, causing you to tune out other people rather than engage with them. If you are angry or upset or worried about something that has just happened or in the middle of an argument or discussion or even if you are totally absorbed by something you are reading or watching, you may not be able to give the attention required for active listening. If you answer the phone in the middle of or just after an argument with someone, for example, the person at the other end of the line is likely to receive some of the fallout – for the first few moments of your conversation at least.

When you are in an intense emotional state, if you can, take a few minutes before you interact with other people. Let the answerphone take the call, go for a short walk, do deep breathing and relaxing exercises or a routine task that helps you to calm down. This will distance you from the emotions of the previous encounter and enable you to focus on the person you are now talking to.

Looking as if you are listening

It is important that the other person knows that you are listening. You may feel that you are paying attention, but if the speaker senses that you are distracted or not really focusing on what is being said, the communication will not be successful. It is important not only to listen, but to be seen to be listening.

Start by giving appropriate attention. We have all experienced talking to someone who says, 'Yes, go on, I am listening', while continuing to look at the computer screen or read their horoscope. While it is true that we can do several things at the same time, and it is probably true that the listener in these circumstances will hear what you say and, if asked, may be able to repeat your words back to you, it is also the case that true, attentive listening has not occurred. The person has not given wholehearted attention. This may not matter. On the other hand, it may. What messages do we give when we carry on with what we are doing as someone is speaking? What do you feel like when someone you are speaking to behaves in this way? Not giving full attention implies that the person speaking is not worth attending to or that we already know what will be said.

It takes no time at all to focus on someone who is speaking to you. When you turn to the other person and make eye contact, you immediately establish a listening environment and, even if it is for a conversation of just a few seconds, the improvement in relationships and communication is vast.

Showing that you are prepared to listen paves the way for dialogue rather than confrontation. Giving attention like this can take the heat out of a potentially difficult situation right away.

Don't fake it

Be careful, though, not to fake attention. If you just go through the motions, your lack of true attention will soon be detected. When you find that your attention drifts and you lose the thread of the conversation, come clean about it and say something like, 'I lost you for a moment there. Tell me again exactly what he said.'

Listening on the telephone

The most obvious difference between phone and face-to-face conversations is that, unless you are using a video facility, you cannot actually see each other's responses. Because we cannot pick up visual cues, our sense of hearing becomes more acute and we are more aware of what we hear. This means that when we talk on the phone, we are very sensitive to tone of voice, pauses and intonation, as well as the actual words spoken. We pick it up quickly when someone's responsive 'mmm' or 'yes' sounds automatic and we are very alert to the rustle of paper or other background noises that may indicate less than full attention to what we are saying. Sometimes we can tell from a person's voice whether or not he or she is alone or there are other people within earshot.

Often it doesn't matter that we do not give undivided attention. In our busy lives, it makes sense to get on with other activities while we chat. We can listen at the rate of 500 words a minute, but we cannot speak as quickly. Our normal rate of speaking is between 125 and 250 words a minute, so there is time for the listener to think about other things and still keep up with what is being said. However, there will be occasions – possibly more frequent than you might think – when full attention is the best option. The quality of your response is very different when you concentrate entirely on the other person and when you, in turn, feel that other person is totally concentrating on what you are saying. The skills of good listening are many and complicated and the whole process of listening, understanding, interpreting and giving feedback is one that requires focus and concentration.

Scene: Becky and Louise on the phone
Louise phones Becky once a week for a good catch-up. She likes unloading all the details about what is going on in her life and knows that she will get a sympathetic response when she moans about her line manager and how her new hairdresser ruined the colour.

Recently, however, Louise has occasionally felt a slight lack of engagement from Becky. Last night Becky asked her to repeat something that she had only just said and was really important and Louise couldn't believe that Becky hadn't taken it in.

What Louise doesn't know is that when she launches into one of her long accounts, Becky puts the phone down and gets on with what she was doing for a couple of minutes before picking it up again, knowing that Louise will still be in full flow. Of course, sometimes this strategy doesn't work quite so smoothly, which is when Louise senses the lack of attention. While we may be able to sympathize with Becky's behaviour, it is not a good example of how to listen on the phone!

The unknown context

When you make a telephone call, you probably choose a time that is convenient for you and, if you are calling people whose habits and patterns are familiar to you, you are able to choose a time that you know to be convenient for them. Giving some thought to the other person's situation means that you don't make the mistake of phoning your friend for a long chat in the middle of her favourite television programme, say, or when she is usually getting her young children to bed.

However, when we phone someone, we do not have access to the whole context of the moment – what the other person is doing or about to do, their physical or emotional state, what is going on around them and a host of other factors that affect the nature of the communication. Even if the actual time of day is convenient, it does not mean that someone is able to pay full attention to you. This is one of the reasons for our sometimes feeling dissatisfied after a phone conversation, perhaps sensing that the other person is guarded or reluctant in spite of their assurances that they are free to talk. Always bear in mind that whenever you make a phone call, even to those close to you, you are invading someone's physical and psychological space and, to a certain extent, you take a chance on the type of communication that will take place. When someone phones you, unless he or she says something to the contrary, it is reasonable to assume that most aspects of the moment are right for the caller.

Listening on a mobile phone

Conversations that are conducted in public are different from those we have when we are not likely to be overheard by people we don't know. When the conversation is on a mobile phone on public transport, in a shop, restaurant, street or anywhere that is noisy and distracting, significant communication is really out of the question. Not only do you have physical barriers, such as intrusive sounds and fluctuating reception, you have the added constraint of a willing or unwilling audience. Of course, this may not put you off, but it is likely to affect the quality of your communication.

Guidelines for communicating using a phone

Here are some things you can do to improve your communication when talking with someone on the phone:

- choose the time carefully;
- be aware of what you don't know about the other person's situation;
- close your eyes and visualize the other person;
- respond as if you can be seen – smile, raise your eyebrows, punch the air . . .
- take notes, but don't start to doodle;
- if you need to attend briefly to something else, say so;
- ask for feedback.

Understand the other's point of view

Listening with empathy

The core of good listening is the ability to empathize with other people. This means that you can, in effect, step into someone else's shoes and enter into the other's personality and state of mind – you are able to understand someone else's thoughts and feelings. Empathy means seeing the other person as an entirely separate entity from ourselves and respecting and honouring that separateness.

Listening with empathy means paying total attention and showing that you understand and accept what the person is saying. You show a level of acceptance that enables the person speaking to go further if he or she wants to, exploring feelings and issues more deeply than they might otherwise do. Because empathy is non-judgemental, it is a powerful encouragement to talk and expand thoughts and ideas. When we sense that someone understands our feelings and is not about to criticize, judge, tell us what to do or jump in with an opinion, we feel that it is safe to continue.

Empathetic listening does not come naturally. Our natural instinct is to advise or criticize or express our agreement or disagreement. To listen with empathy, we need to curb our tendencies to respond in such ways and allow ourselves to feel what the speaker feels.

Benefits of listening with empathy

Empathy helps us to:

- understand other people;
- minimize defensive or hostile reactions;
- resolve disputes and arguments;
- control irritation and anger;
- overcome our natural prejudices and biases;
- create meaningful relationships;
- encourage openness;
- build trust.

Empathy and sympathy

Sometimes empathy and sympathy are confused or thought to be the same thing, but there are some important differences between the two types of response. A sympathetic response tends to be based on elements of compassion and commiseration and offers approval and support. When we show sympathy, we engage in some fellow-feeling with the other person and tune in to aspects of what the person is saying that chime with our own views and attitudes.

Sympathy is evoked when we hear someone's bad news. Our instinct is to show how sorry we are for the person who is hurt. We say things like, 'Oh, dear, poor you, how absolutely awful.' We all need to receive and show sympathy – it is an important part of relating to each other. A listener who can sympathize with sensitivity and understanding has a great gift to offer.

Empathy is a different kind of skill. An empathic response does not rely on feeling sorry for the other person. It doesn't involve being helpful and kind and nice – it is more difficult than that. When we empathize, we have to work hard at entering the other person's inner world, whether or not it is a world that we like or is familiar to us.

Empathizing when you disagree with someone

When we empathize with someone, we allow that person to be himself or herself and acknowledge their feelings, whether we agree with them or not.

Scene: He forgot my birthday

Leanne is complaining about her boyfriend. 'And then,' she tells her friend Mandy, 'he actually forgot my birthday! I couldn't believe it! I felt so let down and he just couldn't understand why I was so upset. I told him that if he really cared about me he would have remembered.'

Mandy does not see the situation in the same way – birthdays are no big deal for her and, in this case, she in fact sympathizes with Leanne's boyfriend. However, she is tuned in to what Leanne is feeling and listens empathetically, experiencing what it must be like for Leanne to feel so hurt and angry.

Empathizing when you know best

It can be hard to empathize with someone when you know that he or she is heading for disaster. When you listen to someone describing, for example, a decision or course of action that you know will only lead to trouble, your disapproval may get in the way of an empathetic response. This does not mean to say that you cannot or should not disagree, but, in order to listen properly and understand where the person is coming from, you need to suspend your judgement and allow yourself to experience the speaker's feelings about the subject.

Scene: Just having a good time?

Shayla is worried about Dave taking drugs when he goes clubbing. He seems to be suffering badly from after-effects and has started to have the day off when he has been out the night before.

An opportunity arises to talk about it. Shayla needs to listen to what Dave says. She has to suppress her instinctive urge to start by telling him how worried she is and that what she is saying is for his own good. In order to have a conversation about this issue, Shayla has first of all to understand Dave's point of view. She makes the effort to tune in to his feelings about the experience of taking drugs.

Scene: True love?

Khan's friend is leaving his job to move to Spain to be near a woman he fell for while on holiday. She is actually engaged to someone else, but Khan's friend says that she is obviously unhappy and he can persuade her to leave her fiancé for him.

Khan's instinctive feeling is, 'He'd be mad to do this. I've got to talk him out of it', but such a reaction will only alienate his friend and shut down communication. Khan's first task as a good listener is to understand his friend's feelings. When he has responded empathetically and listened to what Khan has to say, he will be able to express his doubts.

Empathizing when you have a sympathetic reaction to what is being said

Sometimes we are so strongly in support of what someone is saying that we rush in with agreement and encouragement without allowing the other person time and space to come to their own decision or checking the nature and degree of the person's feelings.

Scene: Should I stay or go?

Nick loves his job, but it causes him to work very long hours and he is under a lot of pressure. He wonders if he should give it up and do something else.

Rachel is worried about the effect Nick's work is having on him. When he tells her that he is thinking of leaving, she is so pleased that she pushes him to give in his notice. She does not hear any of Nick's hesitation – she ignored the word 'thinking' and did not give him any encouragement to explore the situation further. The result of this is that Nick might feel Rachel is pressurizing him to leave a job he enjoys and she does not understand his conflicting feelings about it.

Empathy without words

You can communicate empathy with someone via your facial expressions and gestures. Sometimes we do this subconsciously.

Scene: Smiling on a rainy day

Letisha is walking in the park on a rainy day. She passes a small boy wearing Wellington boots and jumping in and out of the puddles. He is beaming with pleasure. Letisha's face breaks into an involuntary smile as she passes. For that moment, she empathizes with the child's experience and her facial expression shows her understanding of his feelings.

An empathetic gesture or facial expression shows that you understand how someone is feeling. So, a work colleague sits down heavily, sighs, and your body mirrors his slump and you make a little noise that is similar to and acknowledges his sigh. A friend frowns as she tells you about a difficult decision she has to make and you nod and frown, too, as she speaks. You wince as if in pain when someone describes a toothache. Non-verbal responses such as these show that you are in tune with the other person's feelings.

The magic of touch

Touch can be a powerful way of communicating empathy. Just touching someone's hand or arm can indicate that you understand their feelings. Hugging someone without any words expresses a feeling of connectedness.

Developing empathy

Empathy demands a conscious effort to experience what it is like to be the other person. Your job as a listener is to enter the world of the other person. You can develop your empathic skills by asking yourself questions such as the following:

'How is N feeling?'
'What is N thinking right now?'
'How does the world seem to N?'

This is a particularly effective process to go through when you are dealing with a person who is very worked up about something and if that person's values and attitudes are very different from yours.

Exercise: Physical empathy

When you are talking with someone who is expressing a strong emotion – say, for example, sadness, anger, grief, happiness, confusion – observe the person's body language. Look at the way he or she is sitting or standing and the facial expressions and gestures that are used. When you are by yourself, put your own body into the same positions. Adopt the same facial expressions and move in the sane ways. Listen to your body and tune in to the kinds of feelings that you experience. This is a very powerful way of entering into someone else's state of mind.

Listen to the message

Getting the whole picture

The surface meanings of the words spoken convey only a part of the message. To get the whole picture, you need to listen for the emotion behind the words and any hidden agenda that may be there. Somebody may present you with the facts of a situation, such as the details of an argument, but an attentive listener will pick up not only the words but also the feelings conveyed by the voice, intonation and body language of the speaker. Sometimes this is easy to do, when the person's expression is clear and easy to follow, but at other times the message is hidden behind the words rather than revealed by them.

Hearing the whole meaning is comparatively easy when we are on the same wavelength as the other person. With those we know well, we often develop a kind of shorthand of communication in which there is a shared understanding of the meaning of words and expressions. Even in such circumstances, though, it is a good idea to remain alert and listen attentively.

Listening for content

The content of a message is its actual substance – statements of facts, descriptions, questions, anecdotes, ideas, theories. The content is communicated partly through the actual words that are spoken. This sounds obvious and straightforward, but, when someone gives you a lot of information, it can be difficult to pick out the important points.

Exercise: Focusing on content

You can improve your concentration on the substance of a message. Practise by listening to a short news bulletin and see if you can repeat the main points. If you find this quite easy, try a longer programme.

Listening for feelings

Feelings emerge not just in the words spoken, but in the way that they are spoken and the speaker's non-verbal signals. Most of us are sensitive to the more obvious indications of other people's emotional states. It is often very clear when someone is upset or happy. We notice if someone seems to have switched off or is bored. Sometimes, though, feelings are not clear-cut, but are ambivalent or contradictory. For example, there may be a contradiction between what someone appears to be feeling and what is actually being said. Some people are reluctant or find it difficult to communicate their feelings. They may have been brought up to think that it is inappropriate to do so or may not be able to express themselves adequately. A skilled listener will be aware of the range and variety of feelings that may be communicated and overcome these blocks to communication.

Scene: Irina's day

Irina says, 'You'll never believe what a day I've had! It started with a phone call from Abbie before I went to work – that went on for ages, you know what she's like – so I was late, which meant that I missed the morning briefing and so I didn't know about the client's visit and I really wasn't ready. Still, I bluffed my way through. Then Steve cancelled our lunch, which was so annoying, and I felt pretty fed up, so I went out for sandwiches and then I got caught in that downpour. My new shoes are ruined.'

The meaning of every word Irina uses is clear, but it is difficult to see precisely what her feelings about the day are and identify which are the most important aspects of what has happened. What matters most to Irina – the phone call from Abbie, the client's visit, cancelled lunch date or ruined shoes? Does she feel the same way about each of these events?

Unless Irina speaks in an even monotone and gives exactly the same emphasis and expression to each word, she will reveal something of her attitude to the events she describes. Her facial expressions and gestures will communicate feelings, as will the pace and tone of her voice.

Exercise: Identifying Irina's feelings

Repeat what Irina said out loud four times. Experiment with your body language and voice so that you emphasize, in turn, the:

- phone call
- client's visit
- cancelled lunch date
- ruined shoes.

Which event felt the most important to you? Did your voice and gestures become more intense when describing one in particular?

Listening for repeated or similar words or phrases

We reveal our feelings via the clusters of words that we use. You might have noticed that in Irina's account of her day she uses the words 'annoying' and 'fed up' to refer to the broken lunch date. That means this incident has slightly more weight than the others she describes. An attentive listener could pick up on this and think, 'She's really upset about Steve'.

When someone says, 'I'm just so worried about these exams. I know I'm on track to do well, but I'm so tense and jittery that I can hardly concentrate', you notice the words 'worried', 'tense' and 'jittery'. The spoken words also indicate that this person is likely to do well in the exams, but the feelings expressed indicate anxiety.

Listening for emphasized words and phrases

When we speak, we put weight and emphasis on particular words. Sometimes we do this deliberately to make our feelings clear, but sometimes we are not aware that we are stressing particular words and phrases.

Listening to what is implied

Sometimes a person's message will not be stated directly, but will be suggested or implied. Ravi says, 'The car needs some major repairs and we've got to put down a deposit for our holiday. Then there's next year's visit to India.' Although he makes statements of fact and does not use any 'feeling' words, the message behind Ravi's words is that he is worried about money.

Patterns of speech

A great deal can be implied by just one word or short phrase, depending on how it is said. It is easier to interpret this kind of response when you know how someone usually communicates. Listen for patterns in the way people speak. Which words do they use to signify pleasure and approval? Which words do they use to indicate displeasure and disapproval? One person might use a phrase such as 'It was OK' to mean that it was neither good nor bad; someone else might use it to communicate real pleasure. When you are not sure, focus on the tone of voice and the body language, which should give you a clue as to how the person is feeling.

Veiled messages

Sometimes we express ourselves indirectly and do not say outright what we want or do not want.

We present suggestions as requests and ask questions that are really suggestions. When someone says, 'Why don't we get something to eat in town?' it is not actually a request for reasons for this not being a good idea and most listeners will understand this and respond accordingly.

We can present requests or instructions as suggestions: 'Would you like to close the window?' In this case, the listener might respond to the surface meaning and say something like, 'Not really', which would result in more discussion. Even more enigmatic is the question, 'Is the window open?' to which you might reply yes or no, not realizing that the question expresses a wish for something to be done. A non-threatening but direct way of asking someone to do something is to phrase it as a request: 'Please would you close the window?' This makes the meaning clear for the listener.

With people we know well, we can slip into using a kind of code. Someone might say, 'Will you be passing the Post Office?' and you know that this is not an aimless question about your route, so you reply with a variation of, 'Yes, or I could do. What is it that you want?' Sometimes you have to work a bit harder to get at the actual meaning of what someone says.

How to hear the whole message
Use the following strategies and you should be successful in picking up the full meaning:

- listen to the overall statement;
- listen to how feelings are expressed – words, voice, body language;
- empathize with the speaker.

Exercise: Listening for feelings

For each statement below, choose a feeling from the list that you think describes the dominant emotional state of the speaker.

1 'The rest of my family think that I should take care of our elderly parents. They want to push all the responsibility on to me.'
2 'Then he pointed out my mistake in front of everyone. He really showed me up.'
3 'There's this girl I'd like to ask out, but I don't know how to go about it.'
4 'Taking this course has really made me think.'
5 'I do my best but it never seems good enough.'
6 'I could take this offer, but then I might get a better one.'
7 'One day my line manager is all over me, then the next day she criticizes everything that I do.'

(a) resentful (b) confused (c) insecure (d) discouraged (e) humiliated (f) unsure (g) stimulated

The answers to this exercise are on page 119.

4

Ways of responding

When you have tuned in to the person's message, it is time for you to respond. You not only need to hear and understand what the speaker is saying but also show that you have understood. You need to check that you have understood correctly, too. The way that you respond will have an impact on the way the conversation develops – or does not develop. If you respond inappropriately, you could cause the speaker to withdraw or clam up.

What we often do is lapse into a favourite or habitual style without judging its appropriateness. It is helpful to be aware of the distinct advantages and disadvantages of each style, consider their effects on the speaker and the way each may affect the way communication develops.

The way that we respond can have the opposite effect to the one we intend. It can stop people from talking because how we have replied suggests that we are not listening properly.

No type of response is wrong in itself, but a good listener judges when is the right time to use a particular style and can use a variety of types confidently and effectively.

It may be that you employ a range of responses and that you have become stuck with a way of replying that feels comfortable and familiar. This quiz will help you to identify your preferred style.

Exercise: Response style quiz

Imagine that you are in the following situations and, for each one, tick what you think would be your most likely response.

1   You and a friend are talking about your jobs. Your friend says, 'I'm not sure what I want to do now. I used to be really keen to get to the top of the company, but that doesn't seem as important as it used to. My family life matters more.'

You reply:

(a)   'Be careful. You ought to put a bit more into work – your boss will soon spot someone who isn't totally committed.'

(b) 'Do you think you might be having a mid-life crisis?'
(c) 'It sounds to me as if you've got the right idea. After all, work isn't everything.'
(d) 'In what ways does work seem less important?'
(e) 'It sounds as if your values have changed and your personal life matters more to you than professional success.'

2 Your friends are talking about their teenage son's behaviour. They say, 'He's so moody! He just stays in his bedroom and won't talk to us. It's really getting to us.'

You reply:

(a) 'Try to ignore him. He'll come round sooner or later.'
(b) 'It must make you feel such inadequate parents.'
(c) 'Don't worry – all teenagers go through phases.'
(d) 'Do you know what he does in his room?'
(e) 'So his changes of moods and refusal to talk are really worrying you.'

3 A friend suspects that his or her partner might be having an affair. Your friend describes how the partner has started to work late and is taking increased care over personal appearance.

You reply:

(a) 'I'd have a confrontation if I were you. It's best to bring these things out into the open.'
(b) 'This is making you very insecure, isn't it?'
(c) 'There's probably an innocent explanation.'
(d) 'When did you first notice this happening?'
(e) 'So you're worried about this different pattern of behaviour and think it might mean an affair?'

4 Your partner says, 'I'm too tired to go out and have to talk to those people tonight. Let's have an evening in.'

You reply:

(a) 'Oh, come on, it would do you good to go out!'
(b) 'You feel intimidated by my friends, don't you?'
(c) 'Perhaps you should just put your feet up this evening.'
(d) 'Just how tired are you? Are you too tired to see a film?'
(e) 'So you're shattered and aren't in the mood to talk to people.'

5 You and a colleague are discussing your superiors at work. Your friend says, 'I don't know what to do about my boss. She expects me to stay late without any notice and I'm scared it will count against me if I don't.'

You reply:

(a) 'Why don't you tell her that it's inconvenient? You have got some rights, you know.'
(b) 'The trouble with you is that you haven't got enough self-confidence to stand up to her.'
(c) 'Don't get too upset about it – after all, you're really good at your job and that's what matters in the long run.'
(d) 'How often has this happened in the past month?'
(e) 'So you don't know how to deal with the situation. You don't want to stay late whenever she expects it, but you feel a refusal will affect your position.'

'What you should do ...'

If your answers were mostly (a)s, you tend to be an Adviser–Evaluator.

This is what we do when we make a judgement about what someone has said and give helpful advice. If you do this a lot, it suggests that you like finding solutions and helping people. This can be fine, if done appropriately and when you have a full understanding of someone's message. Often, though, people who respond in this way tend to jump in prematurely and, in the worst cases, only just wait for the speaker to draw breath before giving their suggestions.

The drawback of this response is that your desire to sort things out might make you rush in and impose your own judgement on what has been said without really listening to and understanding what is being communicated. Sometimes the real issue that someone wants to discuss lies behind what they actually said. If you get into the habit of advising, it could mean that you listen less attentively, because you are focusing not on the message but on the solution that you will suggest. Also, when we are quick to offer advice, we can give the impression that others' concerns can be easily sorted – all they need to do is this or that and it's solved. This diminishes and belittles their feelings.

Often we give advice from good motives. When we see someone in pain or confusion, particularly someone close to us, our desire is to fix the situation, to offer a solution. The trouble is that our good intentions can have a negative effect. We mean to be supportive, but can come across as superior and knowing best.

Examples

'I get so annoyed with Martha cancelling our meetings at the last minute.'
'You should just come straight out and tell her how annoyed you are.'

'I don't like being single.'
'Join one of those dating agencies.'

'I don't know if we should stay together or not.'
'You should stay together for the sake of the children.'

The responses given in the examples do not allow the speakers to talk any further about their situations. The advice that is given may be sound, but the listener here has missed the point. When someone talks about a problem, it is often the case that what is required is not a solution, but an opportunity to explore what the situation means on a personal, social or emotional level. If you rush in with advice – particularly practical advice when someone is speaking emotion-ally – you cut off rather than develop communication.

Another drawback is that such advice can sometimes come across as moralizing. When we tell people what we think they should do, we reveal and focus on our own values and attitudes, which may form a barrier to listening and understanding them and their points of view.

Children and young people in particular may switch off if you go into advising mode inappropriately. If you give the impression that you, the adult, know all the answers, they may feel incapable and useless and be disinclined to trust you with their problems again.

Why advice is not always the answer

Some types of advice are so predictable that they are ineffective. When a person tells you about something they are doing that is clearly wrong or bad for them, it often seems that the only thing a responsible listener can do is to advise the person to stop that behaviour. However, it is more than likely that someone who is, for example, smoking, drinking to excess, taking drugs or otherwise harming his or her health is very aware of the dangers of their behaviour. No one is actually going to advise them to continue what they are doing. So, when you are listening in this kind of situation, listen for what the person is really saying and try to empathize with his or her situation.

When someone asks directly for advice

Think about the feeling behind the request. Is the speaker genuinely confused? Has he or she made a decision and just wants to hear you confirm that it is the right one? Does he or she want to be told what to do or an opportunity to talk things through?

The other thing to remember is that, even if someone asks for advice, it is a good idea to think carefully before giving it. What if the person rejects your advice or accepts it then blames you when things go wrong? Another possible consequence is that then he or she becomes dependent on you to solve other problems, too. Giving people advice means that they are not encouraged to work out issues for themselves.

Phrases to avoid

The following are phrases you will want to say, but don't:

'If I were you ...'
'Why don't you ...'
'You should ...'
'What you ought to do is ...'
'The thing to do is ...'
'Don't you think it would be a good idea to ...'

'What you really mean is ...'

If your answers were mostly (b)s, you tend to be an Interpreter–Analyser.

This means that you like to read between the lines and interpret what the other person is saying. You have a tendency to tell other people how they feel, giving some psychological insight into their behaviour or pointing out a deep hidden meaning of which they are unaware. It is possible that you overinterpret, going beyond what has been communicated.

Communication is closed down rather than opened up when you put people in a category. True, it is very helpful to draw inferences from what is said and encourage others to explore their situation, but it is not helpful to offer a label or a diagnosis. If you tell someone that you feel shy at social gatherings, it is neither encouraging nor supportive if the listener suggests that you are shy because you are the youngest child or a Capricorn or have always been in your mother's shadow. Some of the labels that we use for certain well-documented conditions and stages of life – empty nest syndrome, inferiority complex, first-night nerves, poor self-image – can be useful aids to communication, but not if they are applied crudely and offered as a summary and solution of someone's situation.

Examples

'The new person at work is very smart. She's got the website up and running already.'
'You must feel threatened by her expertise.'

'I just cave in when he puts pressure on me.'
'You have such trouble standing up to men.'

These responses may or may not be accurate perceptions and may or may not touch on areas that the speaker would like to develop. Listeners who respond like this will not find out because, rightly or wrongly, what comes across is that they are more concerned with their clever interpretations than with offering genuine listening. When genuine listening takes place, offering your perceptions about people's behaviour is a valuable part of understanding.

Be particularly careful with labels that are value-laden. The other person may have a different perception of the word or phrase you use.

Phrases to avoid

The following are phrases that you will want to use, but don't:

'The real problem is . . .'
'This is a typical case of . . .'
'What's behind this is . . .'

'It will be all right . . .'

If your answers were mostly (c)s, you tend to be a Reassurer.

This indicates a tendency to want to be sympathetic and make things better for the other person – a natural response in many situations, particularly with children and those we are close to. When someone is scared or sad or nervous, we feel for them and want to show that we are on their side. However, if we do not acknowledge another's negative feelings, we indicate that we do not accept such emotions. This can send a message that it is not all right to feel upset and can also indicate that we do not want to deal with uncomfortable feelings.

Examples

> 'I'm scared of going to the dentist.'
> 'There's nothing to be scared of.'

> 'I'm worried about making friends at university.'
> 'Of course you'll make friends.'

> 'I'm nervous about my interview.'
> 'You'll be fine!'

These responses deny the speakers' feelings. Of course people need to be reassured, supported and encouraged, but it is better if the speakers in these and similar situations can work through their problems and come to their own conclusions. As a good listener, you can assist in this process.

Phrases to avoid

You will want to use the following phrases, but make sure that you don't:

> 'I'm sure it will work out ...'
> 'It will be all right ...'
> 'Don't worry ...'
> 'Don't be silly ...'
> 'It's not that bad ...'

'Who? Why? What?'

If your answers were mostly (d)s, you tend to be a Prober.

This means that you tend to seek additional information and guide the discussion along certain lines. You try to explore the other person's ideas and thoughts. Questioning of this nature can be sensitive and supportive. The problem arises when you get into the habit of responding with questions and when you use the wrong kind of question at the wrong point in the conversation. The speaker may begin to feel interrogated and threatened rather than listened to.

Too many questions

Some listeners feel more comfortable asking questions than giving other responses, particularly if the questions focus on matters of fact. This can make them feel that they are listening actively because they are picking up on things that are said and giving a response. However, this pattern of response indicates that you are not tuning in to the whole message. When you ask too many questions about factual matters, you may be ignoring the emotional content of what someone has said. This style of response can also interrupt the flow and disrupt the whole rhythm of the conversation.

A barrage of the wrong types of questions shuts down communication rather than opens it up.

Example

'I was coming out of that dress shop on Thursday evening ...'
'What time was it?'
'About eight o'clock. Anyway ...'
'Did you manage to exchange the skirt?'
'Yes, I did. Anyway, I saw Michelle crossing the road and I wasn't sure if I was ready to come face to face with her yet – you know, after everything that happened ...'
'Has she still got long hair?'

The danger of 'why?'

'Why' is a small but potentially dangerous word. In some circumstances, it implies that you are asking someone to justify an action or feeling and want to hear a reply that makes sense to you.

Often there is no adequate answer to this question. We may not know why we behave or feel in certain way, we just know that we do. When we are asked 'why?' we can feel that we are being pushed into a corner. Responses to 'why?' questions can lead to guesses and speculation.

'So what you're saying is ...'

If your answers were mostly (e)s, you tend to be an Understander–Reflector.

This means that you want to understand speakers' thoughts and feelings and also want to check out that you have understood them. This type of response is crucial to good listening, so we shall look at it in more detail in just a moment.

Other types of responses

Judging

Sometimes such responses are phrased directly:

'I don't think you should have done that.'
'That was thoughtless.'
'What a stupid thing to do.'
'I don't think you should carry on seeing him.'

Sometimes questions and comments imply a judgement:

'Why on earth did you say that?'
'What good did you think that would do?'

Responses like this, which seem to criticize and judge the speaker, are not encouraging. They suggest that the listener is superior to the speaker and is in a position to make a moral evaluation of what is being said.

Inappropriate talking about yourself

The kind of talking that is unhelpful is when you wrench the conversation back to yourself, whether it is appropriate or not. If you take over a conversation because there is something you just have to say there and then, try to make it clear that you are doing so and take the responsibility for putting the conversation back on course. For example, 'Samir, I'm breaking in right now because there's something I want to tell you before we carry on talking about your idea.'

Reflective listening and responding

The method of listening and responding known as 'reflection' includes all the essential aspects of good listening. It demonstrates your empathy with the speaker and establishes your acceptance of the other person. Your reflective responses communicate your understanding of what has been said and allow you to check out the

Exercise: Different response styles

Look back at the situations presented in the last exercise. Put yourself in the place of the speaker in each case and consider what might be the effect on you of each of the responses. You may be able to identify occasions when you have experienced this kind of response. How much does each response style encourage you to open up the conversation? Ring a number on the 1–9 scale, where 1 = not encouraged at all and 9 = encouraged a great deal.

Type of responses	How I feel	How much I feel encouraged
listener evaluates	_____	1 2 3 4 5 6 7 8 9
listener judges	_____	1 2 3 4 5 6 7 8 9
listener advises	_____	1 2 3 4 5 6 7 8 9
listener reassures	_____	1 2 3 4 5 6 7 8 9
listener analyses	_____	1 2 3 4 5 6 7 8 9
listener reflects	_____	1 2 3 4 5 6 7 8 9
listener judges	_____	1 2 3 4 5 6 7 8 9
listener asks lots of questions	_____	1 2 3 4 5 6 7 8 9
listener keeps turning subject to self	_____	1 2 3 4 5 6 7 8 9

accuracy of your perceptions. When you respond reflectively, you encourage and help the other person to continue communicating.

We often use reflection automatically. When you listen to instructions, such as the directions to somewhere, you may find that you repeat what you have heard to make sure that you have got it right. In other types of communication, such a response does not come so naturally, but it is often a good idea. Checking that we understand what someone has said is a sound basis for successful interaction. Our personal and professional relationships may be improved by a clearer understanding of the messages we are giving each other.

When you respond reflectively, you prompt the other person to explore the subject in more depth. Sometimes your reflection of what you have heard will point out something that has come across to you, but the speaker was unaware of it. Reflective listening can reveal hidden issues, too, and promote thoughtful discussion and the growth of self-awareness.

How to listen reflectively

Reflective listening begins with tuning in to the other person and empathizing with his or her position. The next step is to feed back what you are hearing. As a mirror reflects an image, so you reflect the words and feelings that come across to you. You give a summary of or paraphrase what has been said, showing that you have understood the facts and the emotions.

Paraphrasing

Paraphrasing means putting in your own words what someone has said. It involves restating a person's communication in a way that shows you have listened and understood the message. When you paraphrase, you are feeding back what the person has said, but, more importantly, you are feeding back what you have heard. It is a vital listening skill and a building block to understanding and communication.

The advantages of using paraphrasing

Paraphrasing clarifies understanding and gives an opportunity for any crossed wires or misunderstandings to be sorted out. The process of paraphrasing and feeding back what you have heard helps you to control any emotional reaction you may have because it makes you focus on what the person is saying rather than on your own reaction to it. You are not distracted by thinking about what you are going to say next because you know what you are going to say next – you will follow and reflect the speaker's words. Paraphrasing slows you down and makes you think before you launch into criticism, evaluation or argument.

Concentrating on the other person's message stops you being distracted, as mentioned, but it has another advantage, too. Paraphrasing also helps you to remember what has been said because you have not only heard but also internalized the message.

At the same time, when you paraphrase a message, you give the speaker an opportunity to put right or clarify points that may not have come across clearly or as the speaker intended.

The difference between paraphrasing and repeating

Paraphrasing is more than just repeating what the person has said. If you routinely just repeat someone's words, you will sound mechanical and disengaged. Far from showing understanding and encouraging communication, such a response creates a barrier.

The skills of paraphrasing

The real skill of paraphrasing lies in using your own words without twisting or distorting what has been said.

Effective paraphrasing is short and to the point. Obviously you are not going to repeat back every single thing that you have heard. The art of paraphrasing is in getting to the essence of the message. You therefore need to listen for what is at the heart of what someone is saying. If you are listening with empathy and have tuned in to both the factual and emotional content of the message, you should be able to give a concise and focused summary of what has come across to you.

Exercise: Paraphrasing content

Which is the most accurate paraphrase of the content of the following statement?

'I'm the only one who keeps this place tidy. I'm shattered when I get home from work and I'd like some help from the others.'

(a) 'You're the only one who works hard and you're fed up with being taken for granted.'
(b) 'So what you're saying is that you're really tired when you get in from work and you'd like the others to help keeping the house tidy.'
(c) 'When you get home from work you're too tired to tidy up.'

The answer to this exercise is on page 119.

Paraphrasing and reflecting content

Being able to paraphrase content is helpful in a range of circumstances. It clarifies your understanding of a situation and can keep a conversation on track.

Examples

'I'd like to work on this project, but it will mean staying away from home for several weeks at a time. Miriam hates me being away.'
'So you would enjoy the work, but Miriam would be upset about you being away from home.'

'I do want to have a family, but work is going really well and I don't want to miss out on the opportunity to progress in the company.'

'So you're saying that on the one hand you want to have children, but on the other you like your work and are keen to progress.'

Paraphrasing and reflecting feelings

Being able to paraphrase feelings shows that you understand the emotional content of a message. It shows that you are tuned in to someone's personal reactions and is an empathetic response.

Examples

'Now that the children have left home the house feels pretty empty. I'd like to move to a smaller place, but it seems a big step to take.'

'It sounds as if you don't feel comfortable in your house any more, but you're nervous about making a change.'

'I asked you to get me a flight leaving from Heathrow and now I find that I'm booked on one from Stansted!'

'You're really annoyed. I can understand why.'

Using the right words

Part of the skill of paraphrasing lies in using the right words to reflect the speaker's feelings. You create powerful understanding when you give a name to the feelings that have come across to you. This can happen in two ways:

1 if you reflect someone's feelings using similar words, you show understanding and empathy;
2 if you reflect someone's feelings using words that the person has not used, you not only show understanding and empathy but also enable the speaker to become aware of what he or she is experiencing.

This last approach can be particularly helpful with children, young people or, indeed, anyone who finds it difficult to find the words to express feelings. Naming a feeling validates it and sends the message that you accept and acknowledge someone's emotions, even unpleasant ones. Here is an example:

'It's not fair. Jenny's really clever and she's pretty as well. All the boys like her. I keep looking at her and wishing I was like that.'

'It sounds as if you're feeling envious of Jenny. That must be pretty uncomfortable.'

Matching up

You need to choose expressions that describe and match the nature of the emotions and their intensity. If someone says, 'I was so angry I could have screamed', and you say, 'You were a bit upset, then', you are not accurately reflecting the nature of the speaker's feelings and he or she might well feel that you are not in tune with what is being communicated.

Exercise: Reflecting feelings

Which is the most accurate reflection of the feelings expressed in the following statement?

'Then they made me wait for half an hour and, after all that, they had lost the form! Then I had to wait ages for a bus – and all for nothing.'

(a) 'You sound really exasperated at the treatment you received.'
(b) 'How annoying.'
(c) 'That must have been so frustrating for you.'

The answer to this exercise is on page 119.

Increase your store of feeling words

Here are some suggestions for different ways in which to express common emotional states. Each cluster of words expresses a shade of the same meaning.

sad	helpless
unhappy	powerless
down	ineffective
blue	useless
tense	confused
uptight	bewildered
wound up	mixed-up
on edge	baffled
pleased	annoyed
happy	angry
delighted	furious
over the moon	seething

bitter	embarrassed
resentful	awkward
hurt	uncomfortable
sour	ill at ease

Reflecting the whole message

Your feedback should reflect the content and the feelings that have been communicated. If you concentrate on one aspect at the expense of the other, you will distort the message. This is most likely to happen if you do not pay enough attention to the speaker.

Scene: Missing the feelings

Gail is watching the last few minutes of her favourite television soap. When the phone rings, she picks it up automatically, but her eyes are glued to the screen.

'Guess what!' says Terri. 'I managed to get tickets for the game on Saturday, so we're going after all! I'm so relieved that it worked out, after all the difficulties we had!'

'So you're going to the game on Saturday,' says Gail, as a vicious argument explodes on the screen. 'What time are you leaving?'

Terri feels as if Gail doesn't understand her feelings. Gail has responded only to the factual content of what Terri has said. Had she been giving Terri her full attention, she would have picked up on Terri's feelings of relief and fed back her understanding of the whole situation, not just a part of it.

Link feelings and events

Usually the feelings that someone is describing are closely linked to the events or circumstances that gave rise to them. We are happy or sad or confused because of something that has happened – not necessarily an event as such, but something that has triggered these feelings. It can be helpful for you as listener and for the person speaking if you reflect back the feeling and what has caused it. You can do this by saying, 'You feel ... because ...'.

Examples

'You feel unappreciated because they didn't thank you.'

'You feel let down and angry because Jim broke his promise.'

This is a useful formula that can help you to focus on and feed back someone's situation accurately. It prevents you from becoming emotional yourself and helps you to empathize with the speaker. As with all formulae, it is a good idea not to overdo it. You can vary your expression while still acknowledging the link: 'It sounds as if Mick's suggestion has left you feeling very confused about what you should do' or 'So you're anxious about how Jamie will cope when he's away from home'.

When reflective listening is particularly helpful

When a person is in a highly emotional state – very angry or very worked up about something, for example – reflective responding is an excellent way to establish a connection and open up the possibility of talking about the issue. When you show that you acknowledge and accept the way that people are feeling and show your willingness to understand what is going on with them, you establish a climate that is conducive to communication.

Children and young people in particular respond well if their feelings are recognized at the beginning of and during a conversation. Reflective listening can prevent a conversation turning into a confrontation.

Scene: Teenage anger

Chloë's son slams his bag on the table and opens the fridge door so violently that everything rattles. He has a fierce scowl on his face and his hands are shaking. Chloë knows that if she says, as she has in the past, 'What's got into you?' or 'For heaven's sake, calm down!' or 'Get that bag off the table!' she will get a very negative response.

Instead, Chloë takes a moment to make sure that she is calm. She breathes slowly and relaxes her muscles so that she does not feel tense and focuses on how her son is feeling. She says, 'Will, you're feeling really angry.'

Will just shrugs, but at least, she thinks, he hasn't stormed out. Chloë goes on, 'Something's really got to you.' Her facial expression is sympathetic. She sits down opposite him. 'Well, I'd just like you to know that if you want to talk about it, I'm here.'

Will shrugs again, then he says, 'I didn't get into the team. After all the practising that I did they went and picked someone else.'

Chloë does not rush in with reassurances that he will get in next year, nor does she tell him not to worry, that it's not the end of the world. She reflects his words and his feelings. 'That must feel so bad, not to be picked after all the time you put in.'

61

'Yeah. And it's not just that.'

Will goes on to talk about his fear that not being in the team will mean that he is left out of the social group. Chloë cannot solve his problem, but the way that she listens to him opens the channels of communication and she is able to help him explore ways in which to deal with the situation.

If someone cannot find the words to express why she or he is upset or angry, you could give an empathetic reply, such as, 'It's hard to put into words'. You may want to move into asking questions to encourage the person to speak, if you feel that is what is required, but don't start guessing what is in the person's mind.

Reflecting positive messages

Reflective responding is also very appropriate in happy circumstances. When people are elated or overjoyed, a reflective response shows that you have understood their state of mind. Other types of responses can take the wind out of their sails and detract from their pleasure in sharing their feelings.

Exercise: Wedding bells

Toni is bubbling over with excitement. 'I'm over the moon! We've actually set a date for the wedding! I can hardly believe it!'
Marion says, 'Oh. Are you sure you're doing the right thing?'
Harriet says, 'Well, good luck. Hope the marriage turns out better than mine did.'
Agnes says, 'That's nice.'
Mia says, 'You've set the date! Terrific! You really sound happy!'

If Toni wants to talk about her plans – both the pleasures and the challenges – who is likely to make the best listener?

The answer to this exercise is on page 119.

Different ways in which to practise reflecting

Once you get used to giving reflective responses, you will find that there are different ways you can feed back what you have understood.

Vary the lead-in Varying the way in which you start your feedback stops you sounding mechanical. You could try expressions such as:

'So what you're saying is . . .'
'It sounds to me as if . . .'
'It seems like . . .'
'You appear to be . . .'
'What's coming across to me . . .'
'What I'm getting here is . . .'
'So the way you see it is . . .'
'What I hear you saying is . . .'

Short reflections Sometimes your reflection can be very brief. A short phrase can be enough to show that you have tuned into someone's feelings:

'Bad day, eh'
'Looking good!'
'Something's on your mind'
'Whew'
'What a drag'.

Vary the style of reflection You can choose from a range of reflective responses. When this way of responding becomes natural to you, you will probably move away from the kinds of formulae we have looked at and develop your own style. So, for example, if a friend told you:

'Dawn keeps telling me how I should live my life. She interferes all the time. Do you know, the other day she answered my phone and didn't pass on an invitation to go to a pub quiz because she thought going out would be too tiring for me!'

You could reflect this back in a number of ways:

'It must be very annoying for you, having her interfering like that.'
'That is so intrusive!'
'You hate the way she intrudes into your life.'
'It must be awful for you to have her butting in like that.'

Exercise: Vary your style

Think of different ways in which to reflect the following statements.

(a) 'I can't make up my mind whether to do media studies or history. I love media, but I'm good at history and my dad thinks it would be a safer option.'

(b) 'I've waited so long for this trip and looked forward to it so much, but now Freya has pulled out, right at the last minute. I'm going ahead because it's all paid for, but it won't be the same.'

(c) 'Harry just won't cut down his working hours. He drives himself much too hard. He's been getting these chest pains recently but he won't go to the doctor. I'm scared that he'll have a heart attack one of these days. Honestly, I could kill him!'

When not to respond reflectively

There are certain situations in which a reflective response would not be appropriate or when you might choose to use it sparingly. These situations include when:

- there is no time;
- you are tired or not in the right frame of mind;
- you want to keep the communication brief;
- you just want some specific information;
- you realize that you are doing it to avoid self-disclosure;
- someone really wants an opinion;
- someone asks a direct question that anticipates a direct answer.

Exercise: Reflecting understanding

For each example, choose a response from those listed below it that you think reflects the speaker's message.

1 'I really want to get to the top in this job. I'm going to prove that I can do it, even if I have to step on some toes on the way.'

   (a) 'You won't make friends that way.'
   (b) 'I must say I admire your ambition.'
   (c) 'Sounds to me as if you're determined to succeed and you don't mind upsetting people in the process.'
   (d) 'I'd hate the responsibility of being boss.'

2 'I'd like to go away for Christmas this year, but spending the day at home means a lot to Lee and I don't want to upset him after all the disruptions he's had recently.'

   (a) 'So you're resigned to putting your own preference to one side because you want to keep things stable for Lee at this particular time.'
   (b) 'You must be really fed up about not going away for Christmas.'
   (c) 'You give in to Lee too much.'
   (d) 'I'd hate to go away for Christmas.'

3 'I'm thinking of getting a job instead of going to university. I'm fed up with studying. I can always do a degree at some time in the future.'

   (a) 'You must be crazy. You're turning down a great opportunity.'
   (b) 'Sounds like a good idea. I got on all right without going to university.'
   (c) 'It sounds as if you want a break from studying at the moment, but you might go back to it later on, when you've worked for a bit.'
   (d) 'What sort of job will you do?'

The answers to this exercise are on page 119.

5
Asking good questions

A good listener uses a variety of types of questions. The skill of asking questions lies in judging the right kind of question for the context and finding a balance between seeking information and encouraging the speaker to continue. Some ways of questioning take over the direction of the conversation, guiding it in a way that the listener dictates, while others work to encourage the speaker to clarify and expand. A well-phrased question will help both the speaker and the listener to a fuller understanding of each other and the topic under discussion.

If we get it wrong, people back away and clam up. Anyone who has been at the receiving end of questioning that sounds intrusive or bullying knows how off-putting it is. Sometimes the questioner does not intend to come across like this and does not realize the effect that he or she is having. You mean to sound interested, but appear nosy. You mean to sound focused, but appear curt.

Asking good questions is a way of drawing people out. This skill, therefore, is a crucial part of the process of active listening.

Why we ask questions

We ask questions to:

- show interest;
- get to know someone;
- explore thoughts, feelings, attitudes;
- find out information;
- establish needs;
- check understanding;
- clear up misunderstandings;
- stimulate discussion;
- get a clearer picture;
- find out how someone is thinking;
- check facts;
- help another think something through;
- help someone come to a solution;
- keep a discussion on track.

Types of questions

Questions can be phrased in different ways to meet different needs.

Open questions

Open questions are phrased in a way that encourages the person to talk. They invite someone to share information and explore ideas, thoughts, opinions. Their particular characteristic is that they do not define the nature of the response. They give no indication as to the length or depth of reply that is expected, so the speaker is encouraged to expand and develop his or her answer. What an open-ended question does is hand the topic over to the other and leave it up to the person to decide how to reply. This means that the person replying has control of the conversation.

Open questions help you to gain valuable insights into someone's way of thinking. Because an open question allows that person to choose his or her own focus for reply, the choices that are made reveal aspects of the other's priorities and value system. So, if you ask two people, 'How was the function last night?' and one replies, 'It was great – the food was terrific', and the other says, 'I didn't really enjoy it – there was no one interesting to talk to', you learn something about what makes each person tick.

How to phrase open questions
Open questions begin in the following kinds of ways:

> 'What ... ?'
> 'How ... ?'
> 'How did this affect ... ?'
> 'In what way ... ?'
> 'Can you tell me about ... ?'
> 'What are your thoughts on ... ?'

When to use open questions
Open questions are good to use when you:

- want to get the person talking;
- want to make the person feel comfortable;
- want to make the person feel confident;
- want to encourage people to open up;
- have enough time to listen to a lengthy answer.

How open questions work with friends and family
Open questions are a good way of getting a general picture from someone. Because the question is not pointed, threatening or directive, you are likely to get a response that, even if it is not as full as you would like, will give you something to build on.
Getting someone to talk about areas that are difficult or sensitive requires careful handling. Asking open questions is a good way to approach a topic gently.

Scene: On being single again
Thea is talking to Jody about how she is adjusting to life as a newly single woman. 'One good thing is having the freedom to do what I want when I want,' Thea says. 'But sometimes it's a bit ... I don't know.' She looks miserable.
   Jody picks up on the sadness. 'I can see you're enjoying the freedom,' she says. 'What about the times that aren't so good?' This open question gives Jody the opportunity to talk about her feelings, if she wants to. Jody chooses to make her question broad. She does not want to put words such as 'sad' or 'lonely' into Thea's mouth.

Getting children to talk about what is bothering them can be hard work. If you make your question too open, you may get a dismissive reply because the person does not know where to start. When faced with a question such as 'Tell me all about it', many of us would like a little prompt to get us going. Open questions focusing on particular areas can work here. You could try variations on the following:

'What's it like, being Carly's friend?'
'What are the good/annoying things about sharing your bedroom?'
'What works for you at the club?'
'How can I help you with that?'
'How do you feel about our plan to move house?'
'What can I tell you about ... ?'
'What would you like to ask me about ... ?'
'What made you decide not to go out tonight?'

How open questions work in social situations
When you want to get someone talking, ask open questions to strike up a conversation and use them as you talk to keep it going. 'How do you know Sandy and Bill?' will get a fuller reply than 'Do you know

68

Sandy and Bill well?' If the conversation is about personal preferences, questions such as 'What kind of music/films/holidays do you like?' are more inviting than asking if someone likes a particular singer or film or has been to a particular place. 'How are you settling in to the neighbourhood?' is likely get a fuller response than 'Have you settled in yet?' In the same way, 'Tell me about your family' is a more inviting question than 'Have you got any children?' or similar.

It is a good idea to keep your questions open when you are in tricky or potentially embarrassing territory. Asking 'How did Jenna's exams go?' is kinder than asking 'What grades did Jenna get?' and gives the other person a choice as to how to reply. A question such as 'What's Simon up to these days?' is more encouraging than 'Where is Simon working at the moment?' or 'Has Simon got a job yet?' Open questions are more likely to make the other person feel at ease and inclined to continue the conversation. Your skills of empathy and reflection will guide you in how to respond as the conversation develops.

Open questions in work situations

Open questions encourage discussion and invite people to express their thoughts and opinions. They are good when you want to get to know where people stand on certain subjects and when you want to gather ideas.

Examples

'How would you feel about taking on more responsibility?'
'Any thoughts on how the new system is working?'
'What concerns do you have about promoting Diane?'

What to watch out for

If you ask only open questions, be aware that you may not get the information you want and that the other person may take the conversation in a different direction entirely. Be sure to intersperse open questions with other kinds of enquiries and responses.

Answering open questions

When you are answering an open question, be aware of the other person's body language as he or she listens. Look for signs that indicate you should finish speaking – an emphatic nod or a finalizing 'Right'. Pick up signs of doubt or confusion or impatience, too, as these may indicate that you have strayed away from what the questioner wanted to hear. You can then reflect back what you have observed, either by commenting on the reaction or changing the direction of your answer.

Scene: Too much information

Spencer asks Ros, 'How did your presentation go?'

Ros says, 'It went really well – they liked the idea and I think that I handled the questions OK. There was one dodgy moment, though, when I couldn't get the projector to work and I thought "Oh, this is the end", but then what I did was . . .'

Spencer is reading his e-mails. He stopped paying attention after the first sentence, which gave him the information he wanted. He asked an open question, but wanted a short answer.

In certain situations, such as this one, you may want to be cautious when responding to open questions. Always use your listening skills to identify what the purpose of the question is and focus your reply accordingly. If you are asked 'How did you think the meeting went?' you might feel encouraged to share your perceptions that it is about time Hari learnt how to chair a meeting and Ginny has got far too much to say, only to find that you have not picked up the clues to the speaker's attitude to the subject and have talked yourself into a bit of a hole.

Open but not inviting

It is not only children who need a little help sometimes. Some questions sound open, but do not actively encourage the speaker to communicate. They may be too brief and abrupt, making response a little bit of an effort. 'How's Nessa?' is an invitation to speak about Nessa, phrased in an open way. However, unless the speaker is skilled in picking up openings and running with them, its very openness may be off-putting, leading to a reply such as 'Fine'. You are likely to get a fuller response with a more specific focus to your question, such as 'How's Nessa getting on in her new job?' or 'How did Nessa resolve her difficulties with her boss?', which are easier to answer and may open the way to further discussion.

Questions put a different way

Some open questions are not actually put in question form. A phrase such as 'Tell me about . . .' is a request for someone to speak and, in effect, is the same as an open question. If you say something along the lines of, 'Tell me about your quarrel with Gerry', the other person will take this as an invitation to talk about the subject.

You can also use statements presented with a questioning tone and body language. 'You and Jess seem to be very friendly these days', for example, is a statement that functions as a question, inviting comment from the other person.

Exercise: Open questions

Identify four situations in which you will ask open questions.

	Person	Situation	Outcome I want	Open question
1				
2				
3				
4				

Closed questions

As the name suggests, closed questions are at the other end of the spectrum from open-ended questions. They do not invite the other person to speak at length or elaborate, but, rather, ask for a simple reply. Closed questions, by their nature, limit the kind of response you will get, which will be something like a brief yes or no. When you ask this kind of question, you are in control of the conversation and you get the information you ask for. You may not get any more than the minimum response, though.

How to phrase closed questions

Closed questions begin with words such as:

'Who ... ?'
'When ... ?'
'Where ... ?'
'How often ... ?'
'How much ... ?'

When to use closed questions

Closed questions are ideal when:

- you want a definite answer;
- you want to agree an action;
- you want to summarize what has been said or agreed;
- someone is rambling.

71

How closed questions work with friends and family

Closed questions do not encourage someone to talk, but they can give you the answer that you need in order to take the conversation further. When you have explored a particular issue, it is sometimes helpful if you draw together what has been discussed with a closed question. Closed questions are also useful when you need a decision or want to pin someone down.

Examples

'So, bearing in mind all that we've said, are you going to invite him to the wedding?'
'What I need to know now is whether you are coming on the family holiday or not.'
'It comes down to a choice between going out to a film or renting a DVD. Which would you prefer?'

How closed questions work in social situations

Closed questions can get the ball rolling, as long as you follow them up quickly with a different kind of question. Keep your voice friendly and relaxed so that you don't sound as if you are interrogating the other person.

Examples

'How long have you been in the book group?'
'Do you live round here?'
'Did you see the play that was on last month?'

How closed questions work in work situations

When you ask closed questions you get an answer, but you may not get any insight into the thinking behind the answer.

Examples

'Did you like Stewart's proposal?'
'Did you think the head's talk was convincing?'

Closed questions work well when you need to be absolutely clear about a particular point.

Examples

'So, did you get the order?'
'Were you late for the photo shoot?'
'What date is the inspection?'

What to watch out for

The phrasing of closed questions can make them sound abrupt, which may not be the impression you want to create and does not help to foster a speaking and listening climate. Your tone of voice and body language can make a closed question sound more inviting, though. If you say a phrase such as 'Yes or no?' in a level tone of voice at quite a quick pace, the other person may feel that you are barking the question at them. If you say the same phrase with an interrogative lift and a pause before or after the 'no', making sure that you do not drop your voice on the last word, you will sound softer. Also, if you ask this question with your hands open and the palms facing upwards, your eyebrows raised and your head tilted a little to one side, you will come across as receptive.

Exercise: Sounding unthreatening

Practise asking the following closed questions in ways that sound unthreatening.

'Yes or no?'
'Did you or didn't you?'
'What time did you get in last night?'
'Do you want to stay in this job?'

Answering closed questions

A closed question followed by a brief answer can make for an abrupt exchange. Use your listening skills to judge the purpose of the question and phrase your reply accordingly. You are not actually obliged to answer a closed question with only the information that is asked for.

You can soften the impact of a question that asks for a 'yes or no' or 'do you or don't you' response by not responding immediately with a one-word answer, even if you feel that that is what is expected. For example:

'Do you think the meeting was effective?'
'If you mean do I think it achieved what it set out to, yes, I think it was.'

This kind of reply gives an answer to the question, but also indicates that you have more to say and are willing to discuss the matter.

Exercise: Closed questions

Identify four situations in which you will ask closed questions.

	Person	Situation	Outcome I want	Closed question
1				
2				
3				
4				

Searching questions

Searching questions go further into what someone has said. You dig a bit deeper, asking for more specific information or examples. Asking a searching question is a good way of making vague communication more definite and concrete. If your partner says, 'You were really thoughtless yesterday', a well-timed searching question, such as, 'What exactly did I do that seems thoughtless?' asks your partner to clarify his or her thoughts and also results in your receiving helpful information.

Searching questions can be open or closed – it depends on the purpose of the question. For example:

'What do you think were Meera's reasons for refusing the invitation?' is an open question.
'Would you be able to finish the work on time if you had some help?' is a closed question.

How to phrase searching questions

Searching questions begin with words such as:

'How exactly ... ?'
'Could you give me an example ... ?'
'To what extent ... ?'
'How many times ... ?'
'Who ... ?'
'Could you clarify ... ?'
'What specifically ... ?'

When to use searching questions
Searching questions are helpful when:

- someone is making generalizations;
- you need specific information;
- you want to get a fuller picture;
- you want to understand more clearly;
- you want to encourage the other person to think more deeply.

How searching questions work with friends and family
Searching questions can deepen and extend the range of a conversation. They show that you are listening actively and that you are picking up topics or areas where more detail would be helpful.

Examples
'Nathan is being really nasty to me at the moment.'
'What kind of thing is he doing?'

'My teacher's always picking on me.'
'Can you give me an example?'

'I haven't been enjoying work recently.'
'What in particular is different for you recently?'

How searching questions work in social situations
Searching questions can be a bit heavy for social situations, but, if they are phrased well and delivered with a light touch, they can be an effective way of engaging with someone.

Examples
'I love my work – it's challenging but enjoyable.'
'What kinds of challenges do you face?'

'It's great having kids, but you worry about them all the time, don't you?'
'What kinds of things do you find particularly worrying?'

If appropriate, stress the word 'you' slightly. This indicates that, say, in relation to the examples, you will share some of your own experiences of challenging work situations or being a parent.
When you ask searching questions, reflect and share your own

experiences as this will create a climate in which the other person is happy to talk.

How searching questions work in work situations

Probing or searching questions are useful when you want to find out specific information. They help to pin down details and give a clearer picture. You may find them particularly useful when people make vague, unsubstantiated statements.

Examples

'Todd is such a sloppy timekeeper – he's always late!'
'How many times has he been late this week?'

'Rita is not a team player.'
'Can you be more specific?'

'That presentation was far too long.'
'Which parts did you think went on too much?'

'I don't think working from home would suit me.'
'What aspects of working from home would you not like?'

What to watch out for

If you use too many of this type of question, you can come across as an interrogator. Also, you could start to take control of the conversation and move it in your chosen direction without paying full attention to the other person. To avoid this situation developing, make sure that you use empathetic responses and open questions as well and allow others to develop their own responses.

Answering searching questions

When this type of question is asked in situations where there is trust and openness and you are discussing and sharing views, you are likely to give a thoughtful response.

Listen for the speaker's intention in asking the question and phrase your reply accordingly. If you sense that the question is inappropriate or it is one that you don't want to answer, don't:

- laugh it off;
- change the subject;
- answer evasively;
- look at your watch.

As you know, these reactions are typical of poor listening. Instead, reflect what has come across to you and give the person a chance to rephrase or change the question.

Exercise: Searching questions

Identify four situations in which you will ask searching questions.

Person	Situation	Outcome I want	Closed question
1			
2			
3			
4			

Leading questions

Leading questions are worded in a way that indicates what answer you expect – you 'lead' the person in the direction in which you want them to go.

How to phrase leading questions

Leading questions contain phrases such as:

'Isn't it . . . ?'
'Don't you . . . ?'
'Haven't we . . . ?'
'I suppose . . . ?'
'Don't you agree that . . . ?'
'Can't you see that . . . ?'
'Surely you can see that . . . ?'

When to use leading questions

Leading questions are a good idea when you want to:

encourage someone who is shy or hesitant
provoke someone into disagreeing with you
make it easy for someone to say something.

How leading questions work with friends and family

Leading questions can help to create a comfortable listening climate. If you phrase such questions in an empathetic way, they can make it easy for the person to reply, especially if your question comes from your empathetic observation of the person. In these cases, you are perhaps not so much asking leading questions as sharing observations.

Examples

'You didn't have a good time, did you?'
'Don't you think that Teresa seems a bit down at the moment?'
'I suppose you're ready for a hot drink and something to eat?'

How leading questions work in social situations

Leading questions can put people off but they can also be helpful if you are talking to someone who is shy or withdrawn. At the very least, the person can agree with you without having to say too much! Such questions can be inclusive and put people at ease. 'Did you have a dreadful journey as well?' gives a little lead that offers the other person a focus for a reply.

Examples

'Don't you think these decorations are lovely?'
'Didn't you think that was an amazing television programme?'

How leading questions work in work situations

Leading questions can help you to draw out someone who is being unresponsive. They can also help you to check if you have accurately identified someone's attitude. If you 'lead' people to an answer with which you think that they disagree, they are likely to protest and make clear their real feelings. This type of question can also get discussions going or move on a discussion that is stuck.

Examples

'That meeting was a disaster, wasn't it?'
'Don't you agree that we should postpone the merger?'
'Helen's not really up to the job, is she?'

What to watch out for

If you ask too many leading questions, you will come across as pushy and manipulative. You will give the impression that you have decided on your views and are not interested in listening to anyone else's.

Leading questions can also have the effect of backing the other person into a corner. When people realize that they have been steered towards a certain answer, you may lose their trust. The other danger is of putting words or ideas into people's mouths and making it difficult for them to disagree. This can make you sound presumptuous and high-handed.

Another drawback of leading questions is that they can set up opposing sides and make communication difficult. If you are asked, 'What do you think of Jason's ridiculous idea to start a smallholding?' and you actually think that it is quite a good idea, it takes a lot of effort to steer the conversation towards amiable disagreement.

Answering leading questions

When someone asks you a leading question, listen for the emotions and the purpose behind the question and use your skills of reflection. This will help you to understand the person's position and keep the conversation and the relationship on track.

Scene: Jane and Sophie go shopping

Jane is shopping with Sophie, who tries on a dress that does not look good on her. Sophie says, 'This dress doesn't suit me, does it?' Jane hears the uncertainty in Sophie's voice, sees the dissatisfaction in her frown and the way she bites her bottom lip and tugs at the waist. It seems to Jane that Sophie is asking for reassurance about her appearance. She reflects this to Sophie: 'You seem to be not sure about the waist.' Sophie says, 'I think it makes me look fat.' Jane says, 'You know, it looks fine, but maybe we can find something that plays up your good points more strongly.'

Notice that Jane has not been led by the question into agreeing outright (not great for Sophie or for their relationship), nor has she let the leading question prompt her to outright disagreement, which may well have sounded over-reassuring and therefore insincere.

You may be unable to identify the purpose of a leading question, so use your reflection skills to draw further comment.

Scene: Performance assessment

Lynn is asked, 'You don't think Ben is the right person for this job, do you?' She reflects back the content and nature of the question: 'Your question sounds as if you already know what I think.' This reply bounces the ball back and encourages the speaker to expand or put the question in a different way.

Exercise: Leading questions

Identify four situations in which you will ask leading questions.

	Person	Situation	Outcome I want	Leading question
1				
2				
3				
4				

Hypothetical questions

Questions that start with the word 'suppose' are an excellent way of helping someone to think of a situation in a different way. They can draw out new ideas and approaches from people and lead the way to further exploration of a subject.

How to phrase hypothetical questions

Hypothetical questions begin with words such as:

'What if ... ?'
'Just suppose ... ?'
'Let's imagine ... ?'

When to use hypothetical questions

Hypothetical questions are good to use when you want to:

● explore an issue;
● generate ideas;
● encourage someone to envisage possibilities;
● discover more about someone's values and beliefs.

How hypothetical questions work with friends and family

This type of question is useful when you want to encourage people to respond to a situation without feeling that they have to commit themselves or they are being put under pressure. Such an approach can clarify problems and help people to make decisions. They offer a low-key, non-threatening way to approach difficult subjects.

Examples

'Just suppose that you did tell Rosie what you saw. What might happen?'
'What if Carly breaks off her friendship with you?'
'Imagine that you do take the plunge and join a singles group. How might that work?'

A well-placed hypothetical question can help someone to see a way past what otherwise seems to be a block or barrier.

Examples

'I just can't go up to someone and start a conversation.'
'What would happen if you did?'

'I can't tell Trudy that her new boyfriend is untrustworthy.'
'Supposing you did tell her. What then?'

How hypothetical questions work in work situations

Hypothetical questions can be a good way in which to suggest ideas or give opinions that may be controversial.

Examples

'What would happen if we changed the system/venue/policy?'
'Suppose we merge the two departments? How might that work?'

They can be helpful if you want to find out where you stand before committing yourself:

'What if I agree to take on the project? How would that affect my current workload?'

What to watch out for

Not everyone can respond to the challenge of hypothetical questions. People whose preference is for factual information and like things cut and dried might find such a question hard to answer.

Answering hypothetical questions

This depends on how safe you feel. If the conversation is based on trust and openness, you could allow yourself to explore your feelings as far as you want to. If you do not want to follow this line of questioning, you could answer with phrases such as:

'I find it difficult to imagine that.'
'I can't get my head round the idea that it might happen.'
'I don't even want to contemplate it, so let's not go there.'

Exercise: Hypothetical questions

Identify four situations in which you will ask hypothetical questions.

	Person	Situation	Outcome I want	Hypothetical question
1				
2				
3				
4				

Exercise: Types of questions

For each question given below, put a tick in the appropriate column to show if the question is open, closed, leading, searching or hypothetical.

		O	C	L	H
1	'How will you cope with these extra demands?'	☐	☐	☐	☐
2	'Do you agree with this ridiculous idea?'	☐	☐	☐	☐
3	'Do you want rice or pasta?'	☐	☐	☐	☐
4	'What would happen if we refused to cooperate?'	☐	☐	☐	☐
5	'Have you finished with the newspaper?'	☐	☐	☐	☐
6	'Tell me about your holiday.'	☐	☐	☐	☐
7	'You'll be finished by the end of the day, won't you?'	☐	☐	☐	☐
8	'Have you got the figures ready?'	☐	☐	☐	☐
9	'What do you think of this programme?'	☐	☐	☐	☐
10	'Is this your type of music?'	☐	☐	☐	☐
11	'What do you mean by "difficult"?'	☐	☐	☐	☐
12	'If I could arrange a meeting, would you be interested?'	☐	☐	☐	☐

The answers to this exercise are on page 119.

Getting the tone right

Not only the phrasing but also your vocal expression affects what a question sounds like. You can create a particular type of question by altering:

- the rise and fall of your voice
- which word you emphasize

Take a sentence such as, 'Are you pleased with the way things are going?' If you emphasize 'are', it becomes a searching question, implying some doubt on the questioner's part. If instead you emphasize 'you', the implication is that other people are not pleased. If you emphasize 'pleased', though, it sounds like a leading question. Your emphasis suggests that you are looking for a negative reply. If you keep a similar emphasis on all the words, however, but raise your voice slightly at the end, it becomes a closed question to which you can only answer yes or no. Although the phrasing of this question is not open, you can make it sound more like an open question nonetheless if your hand gestures and facial expression indicate that you would like to hear what the person has to say.

Exercise: Vocal expression

Try asking the following questions in different ways to create different types of questions:

'What time did you get home last night?'
'Are we going to that restaurant again?'

Timing questions

The timing of questions can affect the way the conversation develops. The right kind of question asked at the right time can prompt the speaker to expand, whereas the clumsy placing of questions can create defensiveness and close down communication.

There is no fail-safe formula for getting it right – it depends on the person and the context. In some cases, a closed question requesting information at the beginning of an encounter works well, making it easy for the person to reply with a brief answer. This is why sometimes interviewers will say, 'Was your journey here all right?' – an easy question to answer that gives the candidate a chance to get used to speaking. Beginning a conversation by saying, 'Did you have a good time last night?', however, may well provoke a monosyllabic reply, which means that you have to persevere with another type of question to encourage the person to expand. At another point in the conversation you could then ask the same question, as a way of clarifying, summing up or reflecting what has been said: 'So, would you say you had a good time?'

The order of questions

In formal discussions, you can arrange your questions in such a way as to help you get a clear picture. Strategically ordered questions will help you to draw out a complete answer. The order you choose depends on the purpose of the discussion.

If the point of the discussion is for you to gain specific information, begin with open-ended questions to explore the broad issues.

Examples

'How are you enjoying life now that you have retired?'
'Tell me how your course is going.'
'What do you think about going to Italy this summer?'

As the conversation develops and you reflect and respond, proceed to more closed questions.

Examples

'Would you like to join this art class?'
'Have you started revising yet?'
'Shall I get some brochures?'

If the point of the conversation is to exchange ideas, you could begin with specific questions to get the kind of information you need.

Examples

'How many times has this happened?'
'Did we get the contract?'
'Did Jack text you?'

Then, as you continue talking, you can open up the conversation to explore the broader issues.

Examples

> 'Any ideas as to how we can stop it happening again?'
> 'How can we improve our sales?'
> 'What are you feeling about the relationship now?'

Pitfalls to avoid

Questioning, not listening

Don't get so carried away with asking questions that you forget to listen. If this happens, you lose any sense of empathy that you may have created. You could end up following your own train of thought and asking questions to support it, rather than responding to the other person's needs.

Multiple questions

Don't run questions together. If you ask more than one question at a time, you make it hard for the other person to know which to answer. In some circumstances, he or she may choose to answer the least pertinent part of the question or the one that requires the easier response.

Relying on questions

If you place too much weight on questions, the conversation or discussion loses its balance. Make sure that you also give reflective responses and share your own feelings and experiences so that there is genuine two-way communication.

Exercise: Right questions, right order

What types of questions would you use in the following situations? Decide on the order of the questions you would ask.

A friend is telling you about a row with his or her partner.

	Type of question	*Wording*
Question 1		
Question 2		
Question 3		

A colleague is trying to decide whether or not to apply for a promotion.

	Type of question	*Wording*
Question 1		
Question 2		
Question 3		

Your child seems worried or upset.

	Type of question	*Wording*
Question 1		
Question 2		
Question 3		

6

Keeping it going

Conversations have a rhythm that develops as you continue to talk. In satisfying conversations, the rhythm is created by the sharing of speaking and listening, as each responds to the other and you share the experience of understanding and being understood. In less satisfying conversations, the rhythm is awkward. You may have experienced the lack of balance in conversations where one participant talks a lot and the other is a passive receiver or when each speaks but there is little interaction or acknowledgement of each other, so that you have, in effect, separate monologues masquerading as interaction. Sometimes the balance of speaking and listening will be unequal, but this is natural, depending on the nature and purpose of the communication.

When you are in a listening rather than speaking mode, your contribution plays a great part in determining the success of the encounter. Your skills as a listener can establish and maintain the appropriate rhythm for the conversation, as you create rapport with the other person and judge how and when to respond.

Showing support

You show support by making it clear that you are listening and following what is being said.

Using encouragers

One way of doing this is to use 'encouragers'. Encouragers are the little interjections we make as we are listening. The word 'little' is important – these words and phrases are short and unobtrusive. Their purpose is to show that you are paying attention and yet keep the flow of the conversation going.

The kinds of words and phrases you might use as encouragers include:

• mmm	• right	• really?	• what then?
• oh	• got you	• go on	• and?
• yes	• uh-huh	• no!	

Encouragers do not show agreement or disagreement with what the speaker is saying. Instead, they show that you are following what is being said and will continue to listen. Your little interjections should demonstrate your understanding of the speaker and indicate empathy – their point is not to express your own emotion or point of view, but indicate acknowledgement and attention. So, when you say, 'Yes, right', you are not actually saying that you think the speaker is right. You are saying, in effect, 'Go on, I'm listening'.

It is good to be able to use a range of interjections so that you can be sure to use language that is appropriate and in tune with the speaker's. Expressions such as, 'Way to go!' or 'Yeah, right', for example, will be suitable in some conversations but not all.

Exercise: Your encouragers

Think about your own use of language. Identify the little expressions that you use when you want to show you are tuned in to what someone is saying and encourage him or her to continue.

Which encouragers do you use when you are listening?

1 _____

2 _____

3 _____

Which encouragers do people use when you are talking?

1 _____

2 _____

3 _____

Matching up

Be careful that the level of support that you show matches the level of intensity being expressed by the person you are speaking with. Encouragers that are either too strong or too frequent tend to put the speaker off. They draw attention to you rather than keeping the spotlight on the person who is talking, as if you are saying, 'Look at me listening to you and being encouraging!' So, if someone says, 'I was a little bit disappointed', and you sigh heavily and look as if the world has collapsed, your overreaction gives the impression that you have not actually understood what has been said.

Non-verbal encouragers

It is a good idea to intersperse encouragers with other types of response so that your attention does not seem mechanical. As well as words, try to use non-verbal signs of encouragement. We are all familiar with the 'nodding head' from television interviews. Someone is speaking, and the camera pulls away from the person's face to show the interviewer nodding in acknowledgement of what is being said.

Gestures such as nods, smiles and frowns, used appropriately, communicate empathy. They indicate that you are keeping in tune with the speaker and understand the messages that are being communicated.

Tone of voice

A combination of the right kind of body language and even just one right word delivered in the right tone of voice can be a powerful expression of empathy. The intonation is important because, if you get it wrong, you can give an impression other than the one you intended.

Scene: Matt doesn't get the job

Matt has applied for a job in Dubai, one that he really wants. He gets a long way in the selection process, but in the end the job is given to someone else. Matt is extremely disappointed.

'Have you heard?' asks Tom.

'Yes. I didn't get it.' Matt's voice and posture show how dejected he is feeling.

Tom says, 'Oh!' His voice indicates surprise.

At the moment, Matt doesn't feel like responding to Tom's surprise. He needs to come to terms with his disappointment before he can begin to unpick why he didn't get the job.

When he gets home, he breaks the news to Helen.

'I didn't get the job.'

Helen just looks at him and says with a sigh, 'Oh.' Her voice has a downward intonation, mirroring Matt's dejection and her face shows sympathy. The effect of this is to make Matt feel that she understands how he is feeling and he can continue to speak in the knowledge that she will listen to what he has to say.

Exercise: The right tone

Try saying the following encouragers in a variety of ways.

	Downward inflection	Upward inflection	Smiling	Frowning
Yes				
No				
Right				
Mmm				

Which combination of word and tone would you use when someone expresses:

pleasure	☐	☐	☐	☐
pain	☐	☐	☐	☐
confusion	☐	☐	☐	☐
fear	☐	☐	☐	☐

Refer back

You show that you are listening attentively when you refer to something that the speaker said earlier:

'You know what you were saying earlier about how difficult the journey would be . . . ?'

'It sounds like the same kind of situation that you described before.'

Giving feedback

This is what you do when you tell someone how you are affected by what has been said. You share your thoughts and feelings and say how you perceive the speaker's situation. Unless you want to take over the conversation, it is important to stay within the speaker's framework and terms of reference so that you continue to show understanding.

Honesty and responsibility

When you express your response and share your feelings, use 'I' statements, so that you take responsibility for your reactions and feelings and do not blame the other person for causing them:

'I'm upset to hear you say that.'

'I'm confused by what you are saying.'

'I felt humiliated when you criticized me in front of those people.'

'I feel disappointed and let down when you break the rules we agreed on.'

Talking things through

In some situations, you will want to use your listening skills to help you and others clarify thoughts and feelings and maybe come to a decision about a course of action. Active listening and reflecting is sometimes all that someone needs to work out what is bothering them or what to do about a particular situation, but there will be times when a little more help is needed. When you move into a problem-solving conversation, make sure that it is based on reflection and empathy and the other person is comfortable with the prospect of exploring some solutions together (Chapter 5 gives some suggestions for effective questions to ask).

Using silence

Silence is not a passive or negative response – although it can be. It may indicate that the listener has switched off from the speaker or that he or she does not know how to respond to what has been said. It could be a defensive reaction, showing the listener's desire to take refuge in seeming to be an amenable listener in order to protect oneself from what is being said and from the possibility of conflict. Silence can indicate an unwillingness to engage with the speaker and may be interpreted as disapproval, acceptance or indifference. When a listener does not respond, the person speaking is not only discouraged from continuing but may also start to doubt him- or herself.

The benefits of silence

Sometimes we shy away from silence. We feel that it is embarrassing or awkward and rush in to fill the gap that we feel it creates. There is such a thing as active silence, though. This is what we experience when we allow people space to engage with their own thoughts and feelings and give them time to think about what they want to say. Silence can encourage speakers to go deeper into their own thoughts and proceed at their own pace. A silent interlude in a conversation, during which the listener displays appropriate non-verbal signals, can offer comfort, support, empathy, understanding. Allowing silence prevents you from rushing in prematurely. This is not to say that you should never respond spontaneously, but waiting just a little time before you reply helps you to reflect on what has been said and gives you a moment to order your thoughts.

Managing silence

Become comfortable with appropriate periods of silence. If you feel very ill at ease with such moments, remind yourself that the focal point of the conversation is not your feelings, but the speaker's needs. Tell yourself, too, that the silence is not a time to sit and do nothing, but gives you an opportunity to exercise some listening skills.

Using the silence

- *Observing* Look at the speaker's facial expression and body movements. They may support or contradict what has been said. Be alert to the emotions and state of mind that are being conveyed.
- *Taking things in* You may use the silence to help you analyse what has been said and think about the way you want to respond.
- *Empathizing* Silence can help you to get inside the skin of the other person. You can observe the emotions that are being communicated via the body language and imagine how the speaker is feeling.

Getting the timing right

Don't let silence go on for too long. This is a matter of judgement as you do not want to break the silence inappropriately, but then neither do you want the speaker to feel under pressure to talk.

You can start the conversation going again by using one of the encouragers we discussed earlier. This minimal encouragement enables you to test the water and you will be able to judge from the speaker's response if he or she is ready to continue. If the speaker then does not choose to carry on, leave it.

Reflecting the silence

You could communicate your perception of what the silence means, by saying something like, 'It's difficult, isn't it?' or 'There's a lot to think about'.

Building rapport

'Rapport' means the bond or connection that we feel when we get on well with somebody. It comes about when there is a climate of respect and trust based on mutual respect and understanding. We have a natural rapport with people who are similar to ourselves. We tend to seek out and be comfortable with those who share our interests, beliefs, attitudes and values and our similarities can be observed in aspects of our behaviour.

Active listening makes a major contribution to creating and developing rapport. The skills of listening are based on empathy and the whole process of listening and responding promotes mutual understanding and sharing of views. Rapport is very like empathy – it is that same feeling of being tuned in to another person. The creation of rapport is something that happens on an unconscious level, but we are powerfully aware of its presence and it makes communication a vibrant and positive experience. At the same time, when there is no rapport between people, its absence limits the type of communication that will take place between them.

How we describe rapport

We use expressions such as:

> 'We are on the same wavelength.'
> 'We just click.'
> 'We are in tune with each other.'
> 'There's just a kind of bond between us.'
> 'We seem to understand each other.'
> 'We get on really well.'
> 'It's like we've always known each other.'

Signs of rapport

You can tell when people are tuned in to each other by the way they talk and their body language.

The way they talk

People who are close tend to speak in the same way. They may not use identical words and phrases, but there is a similarity in their language and patterns of speech. Because this similarity is subconscious, we are hardly aware of its presence, but we do notice when there is a mismatch. For example:

93

'I'm in a right state this morning. I was up half the night after that curry – you just don't want to know! You had the right idea, mate, going for that fish thing instead.'

'Yes, the Sole Véronique was a fortunate option, as it transpired.'

Although there is clear communication in this exchange, there is little sense of rapport or connection because of the major differences in the styles of speech.

Their body language

If you watch close friends in conversation, you will see that their mannerisms and gestures are similar. They will be sitting or standing in similar postures, perhaps both slumped with folded arms or sitting with their heads propped up on their hands, or be mirror images of each other. Their bodies and limbs will be turned towards each other and you will notice a synchronicity in their movements. Each person will move or shift position or uncross their arms or legs at around the same moment. If they are watching television companionably, they are likely to be sitting at the same level in roughly similar positions. If they are having a meal, their pauses for eating, drinking and talking occur at the same time. This is not planned or deliberate, but is an instinctive way of behaving.

How to create rapport

Just as you can empathize with people who are different from yourself, so you can develop a few skills to create rapport in any conversation. Even though you might not be particularly friendly with your boss or a work colleague and even though there might be no chance of you ever getting on well with certain individuals in your circle of family and friends, you can still use some rapport-building behaviour in your interactions with them. This will increase your effectiveness as an active listener and result in greater mutual understanding and improved communication.

Mirroring body language

As we have seen, we echo friends' behaviour without being aware of it. If you consciously do this when you are listening to others, you will form a strong connection with them as they will feel that you are like them.

What you do when you use the mirroring technique is adopt a similar posture and use similar gestures to those of the other person. You don't mimic their behaviour, but, subtly, ensure that your body language echoes theirs. So, if someone is sitting in a slumped position, don't sit with a ramrod straight back, but slump a bit as well. If the person you are talking to makes expansive hand gestures, don't hold on to your cup or keep your hands clasped round your knees – make some similar gestures yourself. Not only does this behaviour help to build rapport, but it also gives you an insight into the other person's feelings. By mirroring their body language, you experience their world and their frame of mind.

Scene: Hatty's night out
Hatty is describing a disastrous night out. She's turned the occasion into an amusing anecdote and tells the story in a lively way, mimicking the other people involved and using her hands and body to demonstrate just how she had to crawl under the car in her party clothes to retrieve her keys.

Des lies back in his chair as he listens. He smiles as he follows the story, but does not show any other sign of animation. Violet, on the other hand, sits forward in her chair, smiles and gasps as Hatty does and makes similar hand gestures to Hatty's as she encourages her to go on with the story.

Hatty starts to direct more of the story towards Violet and less towards Des. She gets the impression that Violet is a more receptive listener. The way that Violet mirrors Hatty's body language helps to create rapport between them.

Exercise: Mirroring body language

Practise mirroring body language when you are talking to a friend. See what happens when you:

adopt the same kind of posture and use the same kinds of gestures
adopt a different posture and use different gestures or no gestures at all.

Mirroring voice patterns
When you match the tone and pitch of your voice to those of the other person, you create a sense of rapport and understanding. When you speak in a way that is markedly different from the other person's, you create instead a sense of distance and lack of involvement. This is particularly so when someone is in an

emotional state, very angry or agitated or excited and speaking loudly and quickly. If you respond quietly, in a calm, level voice, you are, in effect, dissociating yourself from the speaker and the speaker's feelings. Even if what you actually say acknowledges their state of mind, your voice does not show understanding and reflection of their feelings. It is almost as if you are suggesting that the person should not be speaking in that way and, by implication, should not be feeling that way.

A sensitive listener will match someone's voice pattern appropriately. The idea is not to shout when someone is shouting or speak as quickly as you can when someone is talking rapidly, but make your voice just a bit louder and speak at a slightly faster rate than normal. If someone is speaking very softly, lower your voice a little. Responding like this shows that you respect and accept the emotional state of the other person and creates understanding and rapport.

Scene: Rod listens to Drina's anger

Drina is furious with Rod. He said that he would be responsible for setting up the hall for the exhibition, but, when she arrived, she found that the hall wasn't ready at all and she had to rush around sorting things out.

'I can't believe that you let me down like that!' she explodes. 'You've no idea of the trouble you put me to! I just can't trust you to do anything, can I? This really is the limit!' Her voice is high-pitched and a little shrill. She is speaking loudly and emphatically.

Rod feels like telling Drina to keep her hair on, calm down and listen to what he has to say. He also wants to point out that she is exaggerating the extent of the problem – that the exhibition was a great success and they should be pleased all their efforts paid off.

However, Rod controls his immediate reaction and tunes in to how Drina is feeling. When he replies, he speaks in a slightly higher tone than he usually does and his voice is emphatic. He reflects Drina's feelings: 'I can see that you're furious because the hall wasn't quite ready. You had to go to a lot of trouble to sort it and I know you feel let down.'

Because his voice pattern matches Drina's, Rod's response sounds empathetic. If he had spoken the same words in a calm voice, he may well have been perceived as patronizing her. It is Rod's listening skills that pave the way for a discussion of the situation.

Pacing and leading

Mirroring skills are useful when you are talking to someone who is very upset and agitated, but too worked up to speak coherently about the problem. Your role as a listener is to encourage and help the person to talk.

Begin by showing understanding and empathy, matching the person's body language and voice patterns. Then, gradually begin to act and speak differently, moving in the direction that will be helpful for the speaker. For example, if someone is talking in a loud and angry way, reflect this manner of speaking and behaving as you respond, then begin to speak and behave in a slightly calmer way. The other person is likely to follow this lead, become calmer and more able to communicate clearly. Similarly, if someone is feeling very low and talking in a monotone, with hunched-up posture and lowered head, mirror this pattern of voice and body language. Then, gradually make your voice a bit more animated, straighten up a little and introduce some open gestures. This encourages the other person to engage more with you and continue the discussion in a more positive way.

Get the timing right

Always remember the importance of reflecting and empathizing. If you rush in too quickly to 'lead' the person, you may come across as insensitive and lacking understanding.

Scene: Eileen doesn't match up

Justine is bubbling over with excitement. 'Guess what? Kirsty has asked me to go on holiday with her and the others! A week in Spain! Sun, sea, sand and sangria! They won't know what's hit them!' She does a little dance round the sitting room.

Eileen is not enthusiastic about this news. Justine is younger than the other girls and she has never been away from home before. Eileen knows that Kirsty and her crowd drink a lot and worries about Justine's safety when she is with them. She wants Justine to calm down so that they can discuss the situation further.

Eileen sits on the sofa and manages to smile tolerantly. She pats the seat and says in a quiet, level voice, 'Come and sit down so that we can talk about it.'

Justine stops dancing and says, 'What's to talk about? Oh, look at your face. You don't want me to go. You've spoilt it all!' She flounces out.

Eileen did not acknowledge Justine's excitement. She tried to lead Justine to a position of calm far too quickly. If Eileen had tuned in to Justine's state of mind and reflected her delight at being asked to go on holiday, she would have established enough of a rapport to enable her to find a way of approaching the difficult conversation without alienating Justine.

Mirroring language

A good way of building rapport with someone is to use the same kind of language. This does not mean that you mimic a person's way of speaking – adopting, for example, slang terms or jargon that you would not normally use. What it does mean is that you make choices about the words you use and take care to use a level of language that matches the other person's. Don't use vocabulary that the other person will not understand, nor language that is simpler than the other person's (unless you are trying to clarify something).

You can create rapport by picking up on and reflecting someone's pattern of language. Many of the phrases and expressions that we use show something about how we perceive the world. Some people use language that is based on visual perception. They will talk about 'seeing' aspects of a situation, for example. Others prefer an auditory mode, so they will 'hear' what you are saying. Others think in kinaesthetic, or feeling, style. These are people who will have 'a gut feeling' about something. When you notice that someone is using expressions from a particular category, it is a good idea to use the same kinds of words. Doing this suggests that you have a similar view of the world and interpret your experiences in a similar way to the other person. This creates a connection between you and helps to build a good listening climate.

Many of us use a mixture of styles. You could make a point of varying your terminology and noticing any responses to particular styles.

- *Visual phrases*
  'I see what you're getting at.'
  'Looks good to me.'
  'I can't see my way through this situation.'
  'It's like trying to see through a fog.'
  'We just don't see eye to eye.'
  'I need to get a clear picture.'

- *Auditory phrases*
  'Sounds good.'
  'I hear what you're saying.'
  'It came across loud and clear.'
  'Living in harmony.'
  'Singing from the same song sheet.'

- *Kinaesthetic phrases*
  'It doesn't feel right.'
  'I feel it in my bones.'
  'It's like banging my head against a brick wall.'
  'It's like groping your way through fog.'
  'It really gets under my skin.'
  'It took me some time to grasp the point.'

Scene: Wendy moves house
Trisha is telling Wendy about her forthcoming house move. 'It's a big step,' she says, 'and I get churned up when I think about the huge mortgage.'
  'So it feels scary?' says Wendy.
  Wendy has picked up on Trisha's 'feeling' words and reflects her message in similar language, which encourages Trisha to continue, confident that Wendy is on her wavelength and will understand her.

Keeping things on track

Getting a clear picture
The process of messages being sent and received is always open to misunderstandings and misinterpretations. When we speak we assume that our meaning is clear, but, as we have seen, what we mean may not be what the other person hears. The only way we know if there is a mismatch is if the listener tells us so or asks for clarification. One aspect of your role as an active listener is not to take your understanding for granted, but check that you have received the message that was intended.

Being encouraging, not threatening
There are occasions when you need to clarify a point or need more information about something, but a direct question seems too abrupt. What you can do is invite the person to give you the information you

99

want by stating what you would like or need to know: 'I understand that Daisy was in favour of the proposal, but what I'm not clear about is why Justin was so opposed to it.'

Making a statement rather than asking a question can be a useful strategy when you are giving a negative response but want to defuse any sense that you are criticizing the other person. Instead of saying, 'Don't you think that hotel is overpriced?' you could say, 'I'd like to know how you feel about finding an alternative venue.' The other person will then feel listened to rather than criticized.

Something else you might try is the unfinished question. This is when we do not actually formulate a question, but break off and allow the other person to answer:

'And you did this because . . .'

'So it's not that you don't want to go on holiday, it's that . . .'

This is an alternative way of asking an open question, which is neither demanding nor threatening.

Some phrases you could use to ask for information

The following opening phrases all encourage the speaker to say more in an unthreatening way:

'Tell me about . . .'
'Tell me more about . . .'
'I'd like you to explain . . .'
'I'd like to understand . . .'
'I'm interested to hear more about . . .'
'What I'm not clear about is . . .'

Listening between the lines

You may have experienced conversations in which you feel that the important things are not being said. It could be that the speaker does not know how to broach difficult topics or tension and anxiety about the real issue keeps someone talking about less essential topics. If you respond to whatever is said with empathy and understanding and reflect what is coming across to you, you will create a climate of confidence in which the person feels that it is all right to open up and explore difficult topics.

Summarizing and pulling it all together

Every now and then in a conversation – particularly a long one – it is a good idea to pause and summarize what you have understood so far. This can be particularly useful when you are listening to an account or anecdote that is important for you to get straight. Pulling together the main points will stop you from being distracted by details and asides and help you to check your understanding. Checking your understanding in this way shows that you are giving the speaker full attention. (Do remember, though, that there are conversations in which the details and the asides are an integral part of the communication and you will distort the message if you ignore them.) Summarizing is also a good way to keep things going and moving them on if the speaker is rambling or losing the thread.

Example

   'Well, the thing is, I'm going to be late because I couldn't get to the post on time because I was delayed by something I really had to deal with there and then – I mean, you don't say no to Sarah, do you – so that means I'm going to have to deliver it in person. I know that seems a bit excessive, but it really has to be with them first thing, so what I'm going to do is drive round, hope those road works aren't still holding up all the traffic, drop it off, then make my way to the restaurant.'

   'OK, so you're going to be late arriving at the restaurant. Do you want us to go ahead and order without you?'

Helping concentration

Another good use of summarizing is when you have to listen to a lengthy speech or lecture or when you are at a meeting and need to maintain your focus. Keep listening for the main points. You can usually tell when someone is coming to the end of a sentence or group of sentences because his or her voice will become lower and slow down and the person may well give non-verbal signals that there will be a pause for breath.. These are good moments to try to draw together the main points that you have heard. You may want to take notes, if appropriate.

Providing insights

Summarizing can be a powerful way of pulling together the different elements of what someone has been saying. Sometimes when you feed back this kind of summary it can be quite startling for the speaker, providing new insights into a situation. Although a summary is a recap of what has already been said, it can paint a picture that highlights aspects of it that the speaker was unaware of.

Scene: Libby's holiday

Libby and Fran are chatting about their holiday plans. Libby has talked about the process of choosing somewhere that will suit all the family and still be within their price range and all there is to do to get ready to go. She has described how Ray takes at least a week to wind down from work, how he wants to flop around all day while she would rather get out and see different places, but feels she has to keep him company. They need to be somewhere with a good nightlife for the older children, but then she worries about their safety when they are out drinking in an unfamiliar environment.

'You know what, Libby,' says Fran, 'you have only talked about the difficulties involved in this holiday. You've described the stress of the preparations and the pressure you feel under to meet everyone's needs.'

Fran's summary makes Libby realize just how much of a strain she finds this annual holiday.

Some phrases you could use to introduce a summary

The following are good ways to start your summarizing:

'Let me just see if I've got it straight . . .'
'So, if I've understood correctly . . .'
'I'd like to do a quick recap to make sure that I've got the main points.'

Exercise: Summarizing

Choose a television drama or situation comedy – you could start with something half an hour in length. When it is over, give a short summary of the main events. Include what the characters' actions and motives were.

Control your emotional responses

Of course, there is nothing wrong with responding emotionally. Doing so can show empathy with the speaker and, of course, you will show strong emotions of your own, such as anger or anxiety or delight or disapproval, as a conversation develops. What you need to look out for are the emotional reactions that seem to take over and form a barrier to attentive listening and understanding. Such emotions may be triggered by the words, phrases and situations that we looked at earlier. They may also be triggered by your interaction with the other person, as you can find yourself overcome by a desire to respond in a way that is not necessarily the best.

Scene: Tristram lets it out
Bill is telling Tristram about a difficulty that he is having with his boss.

'She changed her mind about which caterers to use for the event,' he says, 'but she didn't think to tell me until I'd already firmed up the details with another lot. Then she started saying that she didn't think the chocolate fountain was a good idea. I couldn't believe it – after all the preparation I did!'

Tristram bursts in, 'Isn't it about time you stood up to her? It makes me so mad, listening to the way she messes you around all the time! What you need to do is just tell her that she's out of order!'

Bill says, 'Yes, well', and doesn't say any more.

Tristram has been listening attentively to what Bill is saying, but at this point he stops listening because his anger overcomes him. He is so annoyed with what he sees as Bill's passive behaviour that he barges in with a combination of criticism and advice. Of course Tristram has a perfectly valid point of view, but this is not a helpful way to challenge Bill on this issue.

Be aware of your physical reactions

Look out for signs that you are getting worked up:

- heart thumping
- feeling hot and clammy
- limbs trembling
- tightening of the muscles
- dry mouth.

Keep calm

You will be able to stay calm and keep listening if you control your physical responses. Breathe deeply and regularly and relax your body. Focusing on what the person is saying will help you to remain calm and feeding back what you hear will help you to concentrate and put aside your feelings.

You could try visualizing putting your emotional reactions into a box, to be opened later, should you choose to do so, at a time when you can share your feelings in a way that encourages rather than shuts down communication.

Employ a range of responses

Make use of a variety of responses. Reflect content and feeling, paraphrase what you have understood, summarize and check. As you listen, use encouragers and don't be afraid of silence. Balance your reflective responses with appropriate questions. As you become more confident about your listening skills, you will be able to judge what is the right balance of types of response to encourage and develop communication.

7

Listening and body language

We communicate using words, the voice and body language – but not in equal proportions. Most of the messages we exchange with each other are communicated via body language. This means that our facial expressions, our posture and gestures, the way we speak, our use of space and distance all say much more than the words that we use. Our non-verbal language is so powerful that even if we think that we are managing to hide our real feelings, we reveal them in our body language. An essential skill of active listening, therefore, is the ability to manage our own non-verbal messages and interpret accurately the non-verbal messages that we receive.

There are some traps that we can fall into. It is a mistake to think that there are certain signals that have specific, fixed meanings. For example, it is often said that people who don't make appropriate eye contact are shifty and not to be trusted. There could be many reasons for the lack of eye contact, however – the person may be shy or bored or thinking about something else. Furthermore, someone could meet your gaze openly and sincerely while telling you lies. You should take in all the aspects of a person's communicative style – verbal and non-verbal – and read their body language in clusters of signs, not individually. Your listening skills of reflecting and questioning will help you to build a clear understanding and check if you have indeed got it right.

Your own body language

Posture and gestures

Here are some guidelines for a classic 'listening' pose. When you are listening intently to what someone is saying, sit slightly forward, but not so much that you seem threatening. Keep your hands open and relaxed with your palms turned up. It will be distracting for the other person if you fiddle or fidget with objects. Make sure that your arms are away from your body, in what is known as an 'open' gesture. You could keep your head slightly tilted to one side as this is a receptive posture that indicates you are paying attention.

Of course, significant listening takes place in all kinds of circumstances – when you are walking or cooking or eating or engaged in a task with another. Be alert to any change or shift in the conversation that notches the level of communication up a gear. You will sense when this happens, as, sometimes without warning, you move into territory that requires a different type of response. Then, you might want to stop walking or pause in what you are both doing to acknowledge the new topic. Be ready to adapt your posture and go into the kind of listening pose just described, adapting it as necessary. This will show that you are focusing all your concentration on what is being said.

Eye contact

You should maintain steady eye contact with the speaker. This can feel awkward at first and you may feel that you are staring them out. To avoid this feeling, just shift your gaze a little to the bridge of the nose or look at one eye only. The speaker will still receive the impression of eye contact. If you look away, you will break the listening connection.

Facial expression

Your facial expression should be appropriate for what is being said. Look serious when someone is talking about a serious matter and smile when someone is describing something pleasurable or amusing. If you frown, you may communicate lack of understanding or disapproval, even if you are actually frowning because you are concentrating. Little nods are great ways of encouraging someone to continue. If you shake your head, you will be seen as disagreeing or disapproving, unless of course this gesture mirrors the other person's head shake.

Space, distance, territory

If you are too close or too far away as you speak, the other person will feel uncomfortable. It will also be an uncomfortable situation if you use the space differently from the other person – if you sit on a higher or lower chair, for example.

Sitting or standing arrangements affect how you communicate. A face-to-face position can feel confrontational, but, at the same time, you need to be in positions that encourage direct engagement. It is difficult to listen and talk if you have to keep turning your heads or swivelling to see each other. Sitting at a slight angle to each other works well.

Make sure that there is nothing between you that forms a barrier. Just move items such as a vase of flowers or a pile of magazines slightly to one side or, if you are at a large desk or table, move so that you are sitting on the side.

The actual territory in which conversations take place is also important. If the space is felt to 'belong' to one or the other of you, there will be certain constraints that are mutually understood. If you are going to have a difficult conversation, it would be a good idea to choose a neutral space.

Interpreting the other's body language

Be observant of the non-verbal messages you receive, but do not rely solely on your perception of what they mean. With all these signs, don't jump to conclusions, but think about the nature of the conversation as a whole and take time to consider your response.

Posture and gestures

Generally, an upright posture indicates a positive and confident frame of mind. When someone stands or sits in a slumped position and keeps their head down, it communicates dejection, unhappiness, lack of confidence. Arms crossed tight across the body can indicate defensiveness, as can folded arms. It is as if the person is using their limbs to create a barrier to keep you at a distance. This can also be communicated by crossed legs. If someone's body moves into this position when, say, you ask a particular question or broach a particular topic, it could be that you have hit a nerve. Feed this back with a reflection such as, 'You seem upset by what I just said.'

If someone's body is turned away from you, it may indicate that the person does not want to be part of the conversation. This goes for arms and legs as well. If someone is facing you but with their legs slanted towards the door, this could indicate that they want to be out of the door as quickly as possible.

If someone sits on the edge of the seat, it could indicate physical or emotional discomfort. It is worth checking for any signs of tension, such as drumming the table with the fingers, tapping a foot or swinging a leg to and fro. These might just be behavioural mannerisms, but equally they might be indications that someone is feeling wound-up or on edge. Clenched fists could be a sign of tension or anger.

It is thought that we cover our mouths with our hands or touch our noses when we are not speaking the truth. Don't take this for granted! There could be many reasons for these gestures and they could indicate things other than deceit.

Shifting position could be a sign that someone is physically uncomfortable, but it could also indicate restlessness or discomfort with the conversation.

Eye contact

When we speak, we do not maintain constant eye contact. The normal rhythm is to look for a few moments, look up or down or away as we talk, then look back. The thing to watch out for is a change in someone's usual pattern of eye contact. If the person seems reluctant to look at you at all, it could be a sign of awkwardness or embarrassment or defensiveness. You need to use your skills of reflection and questioning to find out what it is. Some people find it very hard to make any kind of eye contact, though, so this may indicate nothing other than social shyness or lack of confidence.

Facial expressions

Facial expressions can reinforce what we say or contradict it. Some people smile when they are angry or giving criticism, while others retain deadpan expressions even when they are being humorous or saying something nice. Be alert to changes in facial expressions as the conversation continues. Pick up slight frowns, smiles and grimaces and judge your response accordingly.

Some signs of inattentiveness

The following signs may be isolated or two or three may be observed in the course of a conversation:

- little eye contact
- looking around
- yawning
- checking the time
- frequent blinking
- fidgeting
- biting the lip.

When there are mixed messages

Sometimes a person tells you one thing, but their body language tells you something else. Roly says he's not angry, but he is shaking and shouting as he says the words. Breda says that she is not sad to be leaving, but her lip is trembling and her expression is downcast. In these situations, a person's body language usually gives the true message. Freddy says that he does not find Linda at all attractive, but he can hardly drag his eyes away from her.

When you are in a listening role and it is important for you to understand the person's feelings, check it out by feeding back your observation. It could be that the person is torn between conflicting emotions. It could also be that he or she is trying to cover up true feelings. Sometimes we mask grief or sadness with a show of laughter or light-heartedness. If you accept the light-heartedness at its face value, you are also accepting the person's attempt to keep unhappy feelings at bay. This may not be good listening behaviour, particularly if the reason that you are accepting this behaviour is to protect yourself from having to face the sadness.

Vocal messages

We communicate a lot in the way we say what we say as well as in the words themselves. The volume and tone of our voice, the way we pause and the emphasis we put on certain words all contribute to the kinds of messages we exchange.

People reveal something of their emotional state by the way that they talk. Speaking loudly often indicates strong feelings. Our voices rise when we are angry or excited or happy, we emphasize words and phrases and we speak quite quickly. Soft speech may indicate uncertainty and lack of confidence or deep emotion. When we are sad, we talk quietly, giving equal stress to all our words. A good listener picks up on these vocal indications of a person's emotional state.

Tone

When you are talking, your tone of voice is even more important than the words you use. Make sure that your expression matches the message that you want to convey. If you get it wrong, you will strike a jarring note and risk throwing the communication off course.

Exercise: The right tone

Try saying the following sentences in different tones of voice.

'I don't understand why you did that.'
Say this as if it were a question, then angrily, then in a puzzled tone.

'So what did he say then?'
Say this sharply, neutrally, then with an intrigued tone.

'You must have liked that!'
Say this empathetically, sarcastically, then in a leading way.

Emphasis

The stress we put on words creates meaning. You can change the whole point of what you are saying by emphasizing different words. It is a good idea to stress the words and phrases that are important as this helps to communicate your meaning, but, if you stress the wrong word, you send an entirely different message from the one that you intended.

Take the simple question 'Why did you do it then?'

'*Why* did you do it then?' is asking for a reason.
'Why *did* you do it then?' is challenging.
'Why did *you* do it then?' is suggesting that someone else could or should have done it.
'Why did you do it *then*?' is focusing on the time.

Exercise: Placing emphasis

Say the following sentences out loud, each time stressing a different word.

'That must have been awful for you.'
'Tell me about your holiday.'

Exercise: Tuning in to body language

1 Choose a group of people, say at work, home or in a public place, whom you cannot hear but can observe unobtrusively. Decide what is going on in the group. You could do this with a friend and swap notes about the content of the communication you are observing and your feelings and responses to what you see.

  Another way to sharpen your awareness of non-verbal communication is to watch a television programme with the sound turned off and see how accurately you read the body language you see.

2 Fill in the non-verbal signals that you observe.

	Facial expression	Posture	Voice	Gestures
Someone upset				
Someone angry				
Someone sad				
Someone happy				

8

Listening in challenging situations

Taking risks

Listening is a two-way process in which how each person talks and listens affects the nature of the conversation and the relationship. If you listen too much and are reluctant to reveal anything of yourself, then the listener may feel inhibited from talking about himself or herself. Your communication may even become soured if it is felt that you encourage someone else to take risks by disclosing thoughts and emotions, while you hide behind a listening screen and will not reveal your own position.

Self-disclosure

Sharing your own feelings and experiences is part of being a good listener. The skill lies in judging the appropriate time to express yourself in this way and the appropriate level of self-disclosure. It is very awkward when someone gets it wrong.

Scene: Too much information

Laura is at a dinner party where people have been talking about the latest Hollywood blockbuster. She turns to the woman sitting next to her, someone she has never met before, and says, laughing, 'I think I must be the only person here who hasn't seen that film.'

'No, I haven't seen it either,' her neighbour says. 'But I don't go out much. I can't afford it since my divorce. Do you know, he ripped me off left, right and centre, took everything. I had to move into a tiny hovel and I can barely make ends meet.'

This degree of self-disclosure is overwhelming and out of place in the context. It is difficult for Laura to know how to respond. She acknowledges that she has heard – 'That sounds very tough' – but it is neither the time nor the place for her to respond to the emotional content of the message. In another type of conversation, in which people are describing this kind of experience, such a contribution would be fine.

The safest kind of self-disclosure is to reveal factual information, such as:

'I've got an older sister as well.'
'I worked for ten years in the NHS.'
'I had a similar experience on my holiday.'
'I haven't seen Mandy for six months.'

This is solid ground, with little risk of misunderstanding or embarrassment. When you make this kind of contribution to a conversation, offering a relevant piece of information that supports or moves on what you are talking about, you connect with the other person and show that you are listening.

Expressing feelings

Disclosing your feelings, thoughts and opinions is a riskier step that requires more judgement. It is also an essential part of a genuine shared relationship that is built on trust and openness. You cannot expect people to be open with you unless you are prepared to be open with them. If you are reluctant to share your emotional self, you diminish your self-worth and the value of the other person.

Exercise: Identifying your feelings

Think of conversations in which you have experienced the following emotional reactions.

Feeling	Occasion
Warmth	
Anger	
Jealousy	
Resentment	
Insecurity	
Pleasure	
Affection	
Protectiveness	
Envy	
Impatience	
Fear	
Nervousness	

Shame   _____

Humiliation   _____

Of course, any disclosure has to be appropriate. This is where your sense of judgement comes in. You have to decide if expressing how you feel is the right thing to do and be able to express your feelings in the right way.

As we have seen, good listeners control their personal emotions in order to focus fully on what is being said. At the same time, you have to be aware of what your inner reactions are and be able to identify your emotional reaction to the speaker.

Expressing negative feelings

Communicating negative feelings takes courage. Such behaviour is a high level of self-disclosure and you may feel reluctant or unable to handle it. However, as an active listener who encourages open communication, you will be able to meet this challenge. Just apply some of the basic listening techniques we have discussed. Empathize with the other person, reflect what you have understood and go on to express and acknowledge how you feel about it.

Helpful challenging

Sometimes you may feel that the person you are listening to is avoiding important issues or saying things that don't quite add up. You can, of course, choose to ignore this and accept what is being said. Sometimes, however, you may wish to probe further and encourage the speaker to rethink or explore the implications of what he or she is saying.

First of all, check your motives for wishing to challenge. Being judgemental, critical or confrontational is likely to close down the conversation rather than open it up. Think as well about why the other person's communication is guarded, unclear or contradictory. It could be that the person is reluctant to disclose what his or her real feelings are, which, of course, is everyone's right. On the other hand, someone may want to open up, but cannot find the right words or does not know how to go about it.

If you want to develop the conversation in a helpful and supportive way, make sure that you avoid responses that will alienate or antagonize the speaker and instead use strategies that will encourage confidence. You need to be sure that you can maintain mutual trust and respect.

It is not a good idea to include too many confrontations or challenges in a conversation. By their very nature they are risky approaches. However, as an active and supportive listener, you will want to come to a clear understanding of the person and what he or she is saying to you and this involves clarifying any messages that are contradictory.

How to challenge without tears

A helpful way to challenge is to:

- reflect back to the person what has been said and how you have perceived it;
- point out the issue;
- describe the difficulty you have in understanding.

It is important to speak calmly and rationally, so that you don't come across as accusatory or judgemental. You are not putting the speaker down or criticizing his or her lack of clear thinking, but you are genuinely trying to be helpful and understand the situation. The purpose of a challenge is to encourage the other person to think about the implications of what he or she is saying, not score points.

Scene: The difficult friend

Allanah is talking about her difficult relationship with a friend. She complains to Jenny, 'It's got so bad that I really dread seeing her. She's so bossy and overbearing, I spend every minute that I'm with her feeling that I'm being pushed about and I really resent it.'

Jenny says, 'So what you're saying is that you really hate the time you spend together and you don't like feeling that you're being bossed around. What I don't understand, Allanah, is that, although you feel so strongly about this, you still meet your friend every week. It doesn't add up to me.'

Challenging in this way is very helpful when you hear that someone is fudging an issue or perhaps deliberately not seeing the implications in what he or she is saying.

Scene: Kira's concert

Kira wants to go to a concert on a school night. It is being held on the evening before her coursework project is due to be handed in – a project that Kira has been struggling with. She says to her parents, 'I know you don't like me going out in the middle of the week, but it's just this once and it's probably the only time the band will play in this town! And all my friends are going. It will be the best night of the year!'

Tim says, 'It means a lot to you, I can see that. What about your coursework project, though?'

'Thanks, Dad! No problems. That's all taken care of. I'll just go and phone the others to let them know . . .'

Tim is not entirely convinced that Kira has faced the implications of not having that last evening to finish off her coursework. He hears the evasion in her words and her voice. He says, 'Hang on a minute. I'm not clear about your plans for completing your project.'

This is a calm challenge, which encourages Kira to think more clearly about her study commitment.

Share your experiences

If someone seems to want to talk about a matter, but finds it hard to confront the issues that are being fudged or avoided, you can increase the atmosphere of trust by talking about any of your own thoughts, feelings or experiences that are relevant to the situation. (Of course, you will be careful not to hijack the conversation in the process.) The ideas that you express may well prompt and help the other person to address the topic with more confidence.

How listening can minimize conflict

Active and reflective listening takes the heat out of situations that might lead to unproductive conflict and argument. It helps you to remain calm and not respond irrationally or overemotionally, as well as letting the other person know that you are paying attention to and taking seriously what is being said.

Listening controls your emotional response

In the first place, knowing your own filters and emotional triggers should mean that, when you feel yourself responding angrily, you can acknowledge and control your instinctive reaction, then concentrate on the message that you are receiving.

Listening shows that you are prepared to hear

Show that you are willing to listen carefully to what is being said without interrupting. Phrases such as 'Tell me what you want me to do' or 'Explain to me what has made you so angry' indicate that you are taking the person seriously.

Listening enables reflection and empathy

Having listened, you can reflect back the content of the message. This shows the other person that you have been listening and immediately sets the encounter off on a calm track. If you combine this response with an empathetic statement, you are establishing a climate of discussion rather than argument. This is not to say that there will be no disagreement, but you will be communicating rather than fighting.

The combination of paying attention, reflecting and empathizing enables you to understand the other person's position and identify the real nature and cause of the conflict.

In situations of conflict, empathetic listening builds trust and respect, paving the way for collaboration and negotiation. It gives everyone a chance to speak and be heard, as well as reducing anger and tension. It encourages openness and allows issues to be raised safely.

When someone is talking too much

If you really need to cut across what someone is saying – maybe because the person is confused, agitated or rambling – do so tactfully and appropriately. Use your skills of empathy to tune in to his or her feelings and decide on the most suitable tactic.

You could break in with a phrase such as, 'I just need to get it clear', and proceed to summarize the main points that have been made. An alternative would be to ask the person to give you the main points.

You may choose instead to give small non-verbal discouragers, such as shifting in your chair and closing a file or gathering together papers and belongings. These may be accompanied by verbal indications, such as 'Well, then' or 'OK', said with a downward inflection that indicates the conversation is coming to an end.

Listening to different types of people

Pay attention to the little clues you can pick up from the ways in which people present themselves and speak. Without falling into the trap of stereotyping individuals, we can observe and absorb the kind of information that helps us to consolidate our understanding of a person and improve our listening. If you adapt your style of response to suit the individual, you will find that communication improves.

People who like people

These individuals indicate through their body language and self-presentation that they are outgoing and sociable. You may observe that they make good eye contact with others and perhaps touch people as they speak. They probably smile a lot. Their body language is open and welcoming, creating a sense of warmth. They talk about feelings and relationships and tend to have a very personal response to what is said to them.

Active listening tips

- This kind of person tends to steer clear of challenge or confrontation. Listen carefully for indications that important issues are being glossed over.
- You may need to use closed and searching questions in order to receive specific replies.
- Such a person may not like speaking about his or her own thoughts and feelings, but prefers to focus on how other people are affected by events.

People who like facts and figures

Analytical types give an impression of order and control. Their body language tends to be formal and restrained and their surroundings and belongings are neat and organized. Their way of speaking indicates that they like detail and precision. Unlike a 'people person', they are not likely to enjoy anecdotes or discussing feelings and personal matters.

Active listening tips

- Their liking for facts and evidence might mean that they do not acknowledge the emotional content of the messages they give and receive.
- They will respond best to structured questions.
- When you reflect what you have understood, support your perceptions with references and evidence. Don't say, 'I get the feeling that you don't think Sacha is doing a good job', say, 'From the way that you asked Richard to help with the project and complained about having to extend the time period, I get the impression that you are not happy with the way Sacha is managing it. Is that right?'

People who like to get straight to the point

An analytical person does not mind spending time on an issue – in fact, this kind of person would rather go over and over something to get it right and build up a detailed picture – but straight-to-the-point people like things cut and dried. They value directness and brevity. Their body language may indicate impatience and lack of time. You might notice that, when in conversation, their legs or body are turned away from the other person and pointing in the direction in which they want to be going. Their surroundings and personal belongings, too, indicate that they are focused on results and efficiency.

Active listening tips

- This type of person will have a short attention span and tune out anything that is not to the point.
- Will like specific facts and evidence.
  The body language will often indicate impatience.
- Is comfortable with closed and probing questions, but less likely to respond well to exploratory talk. Well-phrased searching questions are a good way forward.
- Will like highlights rather than descriptive detail.

Finally

A Chinese representation of the word 'listening' consists of the symbols for:

- ear
- eyes
- undivided attention
- heart.

If we listen with our ears and hearts, using our eyes to help us understand and giving undivided attention, we enrich our own lives and the lives of others.

> It is as though he listened
> and such listening as his
> enfolds us in a silence
> in which at last we begin to hear
> what we are meant to be.
>
> *Lao Tze*

Answers to exercises

1 The importance of listening

What kind of listener are you?
1 Yes, 2 Yes, 3 No, 4 Yes, 5 Yes, 6 Yes, 7 No, 8 No, 9 Yes, 10 No,
11 Yes, 12 No, 13 No, 14 Yes, 15 Yes, 16 No, 17 Yes, 18 Yes,
19 Yes, 20 No.
  Give yourself one point for every correct answer.

3 Tuning in to the other person

Listening for feelings
1 (a), 2 (e), 3 (c), 4 (g), 5 (d), 6 (f), 7 (b)

4 Ways of responding

Paraphrasing content
(b) Most closely reflects the content of the statement.

Reflecting feelings
(c)

Wedding bells
Probably Mia.

Reflecting understanding
1 (c), 2 (a), 3 (c)

5 Asking good questions

Types of questions
1 Open, 2 Leading, 3 Closed, 4 Hypothetical, 5 Closed, 6 Open,
7 Leading, 8 Closed, 9 Open, 10 Closed, 11 Searching,
12 Hypothetical

Further reading

Bone, Diane (1988), *A Practical Guide to Effective Listening*, London: Kogan Page.

Burley-Allen, Madeline (1982), *Listening: The Forgotten Skill*, London: James Wiley.

Ford, Janet K. (1990), *The Gentle Art of Listening*, London: Bedford Square Press.

Huggett, Joyce (2005) *Listening to Others*, London: Hodder & Stoughton.

Mackay, Ian (1998), *Listening Skills*, London: Institute of Personnel and Development.

Nichols, Michael P. (1995), *The Lost Art of Listening*, New York: Guilford Press.

Tannen, Deborah (1995), *Talking from Nine to Five*, London: Virago.

Index